STO

ACPL ITEM
DISCARDED

Y0-BSM-450

DO NOT REMOVE
CARDS FROM POCKET

ALLEN COUNTY PUBLIC LIBRARY

FORT WAYNE, INDIANA 46802

You may return this book to any agency, branch,
or bookmobile of the Allen County Public Library.

DEMCO

IDENTIFYING
THE NEUROLOGICALLY
IMPAIRED CHILD

IDENTIFYING THE NEUROLOGICALLY IMPAIRED CHILD

A Primer for Parents and Laypeople

By

MARION F. JURKO, Ph.D.

Associate Professor
Department of Neurosurgery
The University of Mississippi School of Medicine
Jackson, Mississippi

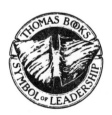

CHARLES C THOMAS • PUBLISHER
Springfield • Illinois • U.S.A.

Published and Distributed Throughout the World by
CHARLES C THOMAS • PUBLISHER
2600 South First Street
Springfield, Illinois 62717

© *1984 by* CHARLES C THOMAS • PUBLISHER

ISBN 0-398-05033-3

Library of Congress Catalog Card Number: 84-8467

With THOMAS BOOKS *careful attention is given to all details of manufacturing and design. It is the Publisher's desire to present books that are satisfactory as to their physical qualities and artistic possibilities and appropriate for their particular use.* THOMAS BOOKS *will be true to those laws of quality that assure a good name and good will.*

Printed in the United States of America
Q-R-3

Library of Congress Cataloging in Publication Data

Jurko, Marion F.
 Identifying the neurologically impaired child.

 Bibliography: p.
 1. Minimal brain dysfunction in children--Diagnosis.
2. Learning disabilities--Diagnosis. 3. Pediatric
neurology--Popular works. I. Title. [DNLM: 1. Brain
Damage, Chronic--in infancy & childhood--popular works.
2. Brain Damage, Chronic--diagnosis--popular works.
3. Learning Disorders--popular works. WS 340 J95i]
RJ496.B7J87   1984   618.92′89   84-8467
ISBN 0-398-05033-3

2252065

A THANK YOU to Deanne Gallagher and Gloria Titcomb for the artwork. Another thank you to Verna Gallagher, who helped me to get the "kinks" out of this manuscript.

WHAT THIS BOOK IS ABOUT

THIS book is about children who have learning disabilities. They may have problems with reading, spelling or arithmetic. They may be hyperactive or hypoactive. They may be a behavior problem at home, at school or in the neighborhood. It is about a special group of these children — children who may have these difficulties because of brain function, or more to the point, brain dysfunction.

These children are not "dumb" — not "stupid" — not "bad" kids. Many have above average intelligence and some are creative and artistic. The good news for parents and children is that they can be helped!

I talk about different people in this book — these stories are true but the names are not. You will notice that some are adults and adolescents; unfortunately, many times we do not have the opportunity to see the young child. It is only when they are older and it becomes obvious that they are *not* going to grow out of it — or that they have repeated failures in school or in their jobs — that they come for help. An encouraging sign is that more and more young children are being brought for evaluation and we do talk about Jimmy who was five and one-half when his mother brought him in to see us.

My hope is that those who read this book will have an understanding of the brain's function as it relates to learning and to behavior. And if your child or one you know is neurologically impaired learning disabled, you will not be overwhelmed or discouraged. You can join with other parents, teachers and concerned professionals in helping these children.

I discuss a few of the things that parents or teachers can look for when observing children that may be important in a certain child. For example, does a particular child have somewhat unusual physical features such as wide set eyes, low set ears, curved little finger and so forth — and what this might mean? Other things to look for in a child are his developmental skills. Can a child of a certain age stand still with eyes closed, arms extended and feet together without swaying, twitching, moving or opening his eyes? How does the child handle a few pieces of paper and a paper clip? How does he draw? You can do all this in an informal home evaluation or "look-see."

In addition, I talk about what you can do at home that can help a child who does indeed have a learning disorder or is a behavior problem. A child's strengths — and these children do have strengths — can be emphasized and he can be taught to cope with his weaknesses. There are other simple "learning methods or techniques" that can be used at home.

But most of all, I would like to see these children identified so that parents, teachers and professionals can take advantage of what we know now and what we are learning everyday.

That is what this book is all about.

CONTENTS

IDENTIFYING
THE NEUROLOGICALLY
IMPAIRED CHILD

CHAPTER 1

DON'T WAIT TO OUTGROW IT

JANE was a very shy little girl. She had few friends her own age. She didn't seem to enjoy playing with others very much. She didn't seem to know how to play.

Jane's mother was often dismayed by Jane's apparent refusal to learn or to practice the social graces. Yet, her mother's friends enjoyed having Jane around. She was "such a good child, so quiet and no trouble at all."

Miss Brown, a neighbor and kindergarten teacher, thought Jane was unusually smart for her age. She encouraged Jane's parents to start her in kindergarten at four years of age. Jane remembers this as almost an out-of-body experience. She says she felt as if she were on the outside looking in, never quite part of what was going on even when going through the motions.

A very thin child, Jane doesn't remember ever feeling really hungry. When local school law required that she have a physical examination before starting first grade, she remembers the results as being traumatic. The doctor told her mother, a nutrition buff, that Jane could not start first grade unless she gained at least five pounds. Her mother was insulted, interpreting this as meaning she didn't take care of her child properly.

Nevertheless, a weight gain program began and continued throughout her school years. Meals became a battle; force feeding was the battle plan. Jane reacted as other members of her family did to stress: chronic indigestion, nausea under any kind of stress, vomiting when she tried to eat under stressful situations. These

3

symptoms continue to this day.

Jane did gain enough weight to begin first grade. She did quite well scholastically. She was often "teacher's pet," but she continued to be stand-offish with her peers. She continued to do well until the fourth grade.

During the fourth grade, however, the family's moves necessitated three changes in schools for Jane. As she began to show academic problems, they were attributed to the difficulty in adjusting to those changes. She was encouraged to try harder, make new friends, get used to the changes.

Jane remembers this period differently. She didn't like to move, but she was aware that she couldn't memorize the multiplication tables. As arithmetic problems became more difficult—there were columns of figures to add, subtraction involved double digit numbers, division was more than just reversing the multiplication process—her grades began to reflect serious problems. Again, the answer was, "try harder."

That same year, memory work involved reciting poems and taking history tests. Jane understood material as it was discussed in class. She knew where to look for information if she needed it later. But, the memorization for recitation and testing was agony. When asked to provide names, dates and places, she couldn't.

Jane was always the last chosen for any athletic team. She was somewhat clumsy and uncoordinated. She often cried over what she perceived as a lack of popularity. Eventually, she found many excuses not to participate. This problem and these excuses continued through her second year in college.

Parents and teachers always had the same appraisal of Jane's shortcomings. "You're a very smart girl. There's absolutely no reason why you can't do these things. You're just not trying." No amount of, "I *am* trying," appeased the adults in Jane's life.

Jane now remembers her childhood as "always feeling lonely, always at least a little depressed." She didn't know the meaning of the words at the time. She assumed everyone else felt the same way. The only times she felt somewhat at peace were behind the closed doors of her bedroom.

To entertain herself, she began drawing very early. She would spend hours copying drawings in children's books. As early as she could, she took up letter writing. Letters to absent relatives might be ten or twelve pages long. Each would be in a different "fancy" handwriting. The drawings were considered cute; the letters were often ignored because she "answered them too soon and wrote too much."

Jane's shyness, lack of athletic ability and difficulty with school work continued through high school and two years of college. While she participated in those extracurricular activities that allowed her to work by herself, illustrating or writing for the school newspaper, she rarely dated or attended school social functions.

She married the first man who asked her, secretly afraid no one else would. Her marriage lasted longer than most other associations, but it ended after twenty years. As an adult, if a friendship or a job didn't suit her, she would withdraw without any hesitation. The stress of a number of jobs resulted in resignations, sometimes hasty and in a fit of temper.

At fifty, she quit her last secretarial job, considered herself a total failure at everything, and experienced a long period of severe depression. After six months of seemingly fruitless therapy, it was suggested that something physical might be involved. Surely the depression would have improved in that time if only emotions were involved. It was at this point that I met Jane. We'll continue with her story later.

About the same time that I met Jane, a juvenile court judge referred a teenage boy to me. Ray was just two months short of being legally classified as an adult. He had been in and out of serious trouble for a number of years. His history of trouble making went back to early grade school.

When Ray's mother brought him to my office, she told me that they had moved to this area only recently. They had, in fact, moved here in one last ditch attempt to give Ray a new start. Their hope had been that new associations and an unprejudiced school situation would help turn things around.

Ray's intolerable behavior had begun in the early elementary grades. By the time he was in third grade, it was so bad that he was referred to a child psychologist. Despite his parents' best efforts to follow the prescription of firmness, consistency and structure, his hyperactivity could not be controlled. The father worried about Ray to the point of making daily visits to the school to reassure Ray that he was loved and to give reinforcement for good behavior.

As he moved on in school, Ray continued to be difficult to get along with. He often deliberately aggravated classmates. He did put some energy into playing football, seemingly a good way to work off excessive energy. He was pretty good at it and never seemed to feel pain when injured. His total body movement seemed to be coordinated well enough for sports, but his hands had trouble with anything requiring finer movement. His handwriting and drawing were exceptionally poor, even "for a boy."

Serious trouble began in high school. He became involved in various kinds of destructive behavior. He used marijuana and other drugs. He couldn't handle alcohol at all, becoming violent and assaulting others. Once he drove his fist through a wall and broke furniture. In one year, he had several automobile accidents. He became a regular in the local juvenile court. He spent time in juvenile detention centers and in halfway houses. He picked up the same type of friends and activities after moving to this area. It was not long before he was back in court again. This judge referred him to us for testing, the first time this approach had been taken.

All Ray's problems had cost the family a lot in both frustration and money. The father had a position that would normally allow the mother to stay home with the four children. Instead, the mother had to go to work to help pay for all the legal fees, restitution, fines, etc. involved with Ray's textbook example of apparently sociopathic behavior. At one time, they started a business of their own. This was designed to let Ray's mother have a little more time with the children and to provide a place for Ray and the other children to work, to earn some money of their own. Ray's expenses were so great, the business couldn't support them.

When Ray's father talked about all their experiences, he said, "We're 'abused parents.' We're not just afraid of what is going to happen to him, we're afraid for our own physical safety. I am not an old man, but when Ray becomes violent at home, I cannot restrain him. The whole family is in danger. Ray has dropped out of school. We don't know where he is or what to expect at any time."

Take a few minutes and think about these two people. Can you see any similarities?

If you had Jane in your classroom today, would you recognize that she had a problem? What would you do about it? What do you think would have helped her most? I'm sure you have more immediate and profound reactions to Ray's story. How would you have handled him? Beyond the help his parents tried to get for him, what would you have done?

Although these two people appear so different, they do have something in common — brain dysfunction.

CHAPTER 2

WHAT'S GOING ON HERE?

BRAIN dysfunction

That's a scary term even when you don't know what it means. It can be more frightening if you first learn about it as it applies to someone you love. Yet, it is something that can be dealt with in a productive way once diagnosed. If it is diagnosed in children at an early age, the possibilities for a fruitful life are much greater.

There are many other terms that mean approximately the same thing as brain dysfunction: altered neurological status, compromised brain function, impaired brain function, brain related disability, brain based disability, neurological impairment, etc. Just for variety, I may use some of these other terms as I describe the problem. None of them are any less frightening than others. Whatever you choose to call it, there are greater and lesser degrees of impairment. Jane's is a relatively mild example; Ray's serious to the extreme.

Jane is fifty, Ray is almost eighteen. When they were small children, we didn't know much about brain dysfunction. We couldn't recognize it as such, especially if disguised as something else. We couldn't do a whole lot to help.

With the information we now have available, we can diagnose better and offer a number of kinds of remediation. Children with brain dysfunction need not go through life feeling dumb, unpopular or unsuccessful. They need not drop out of school to become, perhaps our chronically unemployed welfare cases, our juvenile delinquents or our unwed mothers in the frustrated attempt to cope with their unrecognized disorder.

This book is for concerned parents. It's for our present and future teachers in preschools and early elementary grades. Pediatricians and child psychologists also need this information. I list these groups in, what seems to me, their order of importance to children.

Obviously, it's the parents who are with their children in the earliest years. If they see unusual behavior before their children reach school age, they need to know to what degree they are out of the ordinary. Teachers are the next most important people in children's lives. They are the first to see children in groups of the same approximate age on a continuing basis. Almost without thinking, they habitually compare children with each other. This happens above and beyond what is required for academic purposes.

I believe parents and teachers themselves might be able to alert pediatricians and child psychologists to the possibility of brain dysfunction in certain of their children. Neither of these professional groups can possibly know all of the symptoms as they exist in a child unless the parents and teachers can tell them the whole story.

It is unfortunate but most of the research and resulting discoveries about neurological impairments have been kept within the ranks of academic institutions. It has not necessarily been a deliberate attempt to keep secrets. To the contrary, much has been written on the subject. But, it has been written in such a manner that few would just pick it up and read it. Pediatricians, for instance, are extremely busy. Most of the time, they must be concerned with an immediate medical crisis or procedure. Often, they don't have time to seek out information that doesn't seem to be of medical importance, that does not seem to have any bearing on what is being treated at the moment. Psychologists don't usually see a child until the emotional and educational problems that accompany brain dysfunction have shown themselves. The two professions do not necessarily compare information with each other. This book is my attempt to get all the people concerned with a child's future working together.

Let's talk about some things we see in children all the time before we go into detail about brain dysfunction itself. These are things all of us have heard about and may be considered to fall within the so-called normal range of variation.

We all know there are many variations in children. They come in different sizes and builds even though they may have the same birth dates. Some are naturally left handed. Some are perfect angels, others are terrible brats. Some learn a little faster, others have more trouble with one subject than others.

Teachers and some parents are aware of learning difficulties. Children with these disabilities may have normal, above average or even superior intelligence. Yet, for one reason or another, they have unusual difficulty learning certain types of material.

I emphasize the fact that many children with learning difficulties have above average or superior intelligence. These children are not "dumb." Their nursery and kindergarten teachers, as Jane's, considered them "as smart for their age." They are not "refusing to try." They are putting just as much effort into their learning as any other child. They may be exceptionally good at other types of material or activities. Sometimes, they just need a different way to approach the subject. In other situations, it might be well to encourage the child to build up skills in other areas in which he does better once he has learned the basics of what is, to him, a difficult subject.

When it comes to behavior, I guess you hear more about *hyperactive* behavior from teachers than from anybody else. When they talk about children with this disorder, they are usually moaning and groaning. That's not surprising. Such impulsive and uncontrollable children can make chaos out of the simplest classroom activity. Ray was one of these children.

At the other end of the behavior scale, though, are children who ask for and get little attention. Jane is a good example of this. These children cause no obvious or immediate problems in class. They are seldom mentioned. They could be called the classroom wallflowers. So quiet they are hardly noticed, their seemingly good behavior later becomes their undoing. Much too late, it may be discovered that they have not acquired skills necessary to perform as self-supporting, productive adults. These are the *hypoactive* children. Hyperactive. Hypoactive. Opposite ends of the pole.

Let's make a very clear distinction. Children may have a learning disability and not be behavior problems. Children can be hyperactive or hypoactive and and not have a learning disability. It is possible to have either or both and not have a brain dysfunction. But, the chances are that if they have *both* there may be a problem inside the brain. We must be extremely careful, however, not to draw conclusions too quickly or to apply the term on the basis of inadequate knowledge.

My concern is with those children who have both learning and behavior problems PLUS a number of physical signs and symptoms. It's the combination of all these things which indicates testing and evaluation may be appropriate to confirm or eliminate the possibility of a brain-based impairment. I repeat this *combination* premise throughout the book because it is very important when a parent or teacher is seeking to identify a child who needs our help.

Probably the most important reason to note signs and symptoms in preschool and early grade school children, is that the "He'll grow out of it" approach may be asking for much greater misery down the road. True, the impairment can and may improve with age, but most of the time a cure cannot happen. Even with medication or re-mediation, a cure, as such, won't happen. But, we can teach the child to circumvent, compensate, accommodate or control the manifestations of the dysfunction. Medication may be suggested, for a time, but other training may also be appropriate.

Early detection is extremely important to the child's future; yet I cnnot make an expert diagnostician out of you in a small book. What I can do is give you some information so that you will know what to call to the attention of experts in the field.

Not all children can compensate as well as Jane did, for as many years, with no outside help. Neither do all children develop into such serious problems for society as Ray did. The Jane's and Ray's of today need not lead unsatisfactory lives. We now know there are reasons and answers for their distress.

What is brain dysfunction?

Simply put, it is the inability of any part or parts of the brain to operate with certain standards for any number of reasons. Since many areas of the brain have certain functions, the dysfunction of one or more can cause different types of learning or behavioral problems.

Brain dysfunction does not mean the entire brain is nonfunctional. It seems a little less frightening if you compare this problem with one your car might have. If your spark plugs are worn or dirty, your car may not operate properly. But you can correct the problem by cleaning the plugs or replacing them. A more personal example might be that if your arm is broken, the rest of your body is still functioning despite extreme discomfort in one place.

We can't replace brain parts yet, but we can circumvent or retrain impaired areas to accommodate for the difficulties. Jane's instincts led her to build up skills in areas where she could excel. She took art and journalism courses when she could. As a result, she edited several corporate in-house newspapers. At times, she sold paintings. Her organizational skills are excellent and she has little difficulty finding places where she can use them. Had all these skills been recognized and fostered earlier, she might have done even more with her talents.

What causes brain dysfunction?

I doubt that we know all the causes yet, but we'll start talking about the ones you've read about or seen.

Nearly all of us know of someone who has had a stroke. The seriousness of the stroke depends upon what area of the brain has been affected, and how much damage has been done. Some patients may be mildly affected and can resume normal activities. Others have difficulty speaking, remembering or moving. If the brain has been affected on the left side, the right side of the body may be immobile.

We've all read and heard about the attempted assassination of President Reagan. We know that his press secretary, Mr. James Brady, was shot in the head at the same time. This injury caused some brain dysfunction that kept Mr. Brady away from his office duties for many months. Even now, although he is able to work some, he continues to suffer the results of that brain injury. He will continue to have problems for a long time. No one knows how much he will be able to do in the future but he will continue to have special help in overcoming the damage.

Of course, some children suffer head injuries as they grow up. When experience tells us that there may be brain dysfunction, we run an electroencephalogram — EEG or brain wave test — to see what, if any, abnormality is present.

Strips from three EEG tracings are shown in Figure 1 to give you an idea of what an EEG tracing looks like. All three EEGs are abnormal. They were taken from a father, the tracing on the right, and two of his children. Their story will be told later.

EEG tracings really do look like chicken scratchings to most people. The recordings are made by attaching sensors or electrodes to

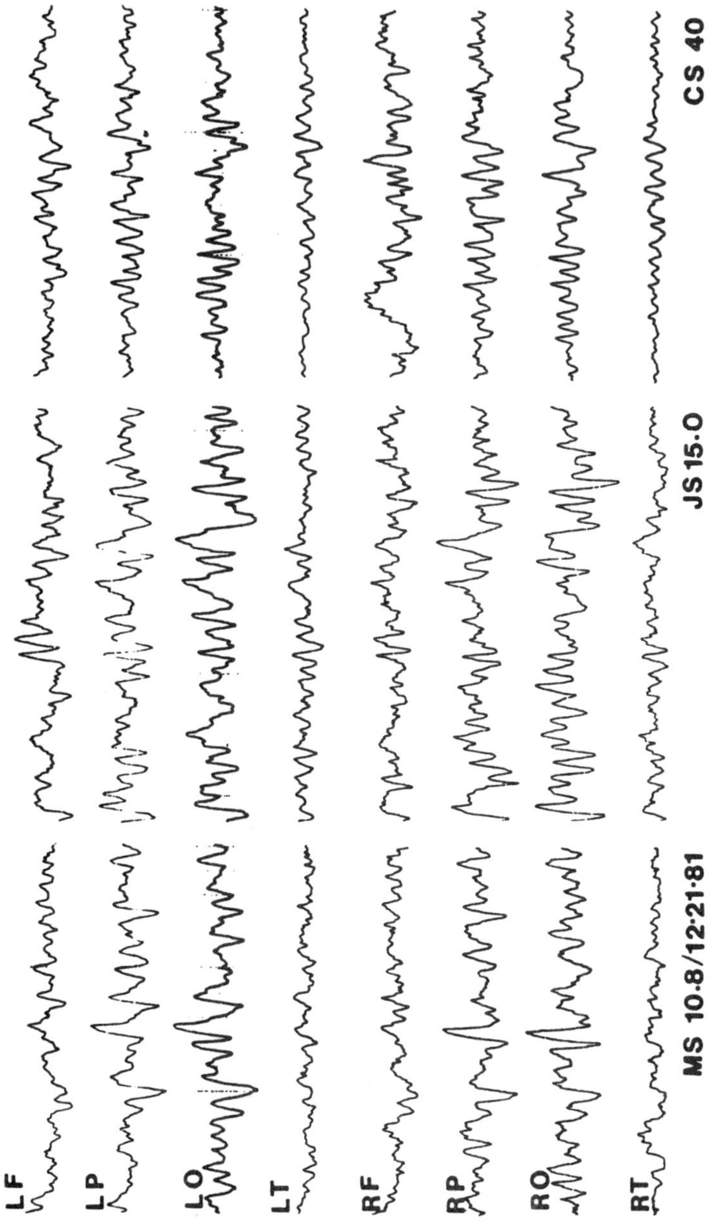

Figure 1.

eight different areas of the scalp. As these sensors pick up electrical activity from the brain, the machine records it on eight lines, one for each sensor, the first four recording the activity of the left brain and the last four the right brain. One or more of these wiggly lines can be abnormal.

There is a new instrument, a magnetoencephalogram, which can pinpoint activity in and outside the brain cells as it detects and records the magnetic fields produced by the electrical activity. The EEG is limited to recording activity outside the cells. This instrument is proving to be useful in pinpointing small areas of the brain which may be malfunctioning.

Occasionally, a child is born with an obvious and immediate problem. The head is greatly enlarged by hydrocephalus (water on the brain). The fluids necessary for proper brain function cannot circulate or drain as they should. Consequently, they stay dammed up in the ventricles—hollow spaces in the middle of the brain—and cause swelling. In this situation, a CAT scan will show the enlarged ventricles. The excessive pressure caused by this lack of circulation can injure surrounding brain tissue.

The next illustration (Fig. 2) shows what a CAT scan looks like. It's actually a series of x-ray pictures, each of a slightly different layer of the brain. These pictures are then assembled by a computer—and you then have a composite of that level of the brain. This scan is of the brain of a one-year-old child with meningitis. The ventricles— the dark shapes in the middle—are greatly enlarged because of too much pressure on the inside of the infant's brain.

Injuries to the brain may occur at birth. Sometimes the use of forceps during delivery creates problems. An unduly long labor can be a factor in brain dysfunction. Even in a normal delivery, the brain—especially the side areas of the brain above the ears—can be damaged by its own housing, the skull. The inside of the skull in this region has many tiny, rough projections that can scrape the surface of the baby's brain. Simply being born can be hazardous to the health.

At least two other causes of brain dysfunction are not so readily apparent. One is genetic or hereditary in origin. The other results from some kind of interruption in the course of fetal development.

Naturally, we take family histories when we see a child. As we ask more and more questions about the child, a parent will say, "Oh,

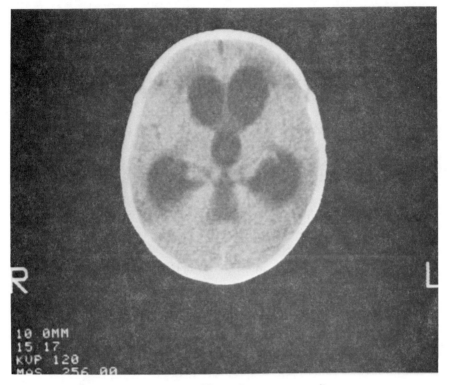

Figure 2.

yes! I do that," or "My mother acted that way." Occasionally, the parents will ask that we run an EEG on them or ask that the other children in the family be tested too. Within limits, we can tell whether an abnormality is genetic or acquired, such as early brain insult.

Also, I'll go into it in more detail later on, developmental "error" can be sometimes suggested by an unusual physical feature of the head, hands or feet, for instance.

Knowledge of probable cause of brain dysfunction, such as early brain damage or genetic factors may help us determine what kind of remediation to use.

Marilyn is another excellent example of an unrecognized brain dysfunction. Apparently, no one even noticed that she had a learning disability, much less other symptoms of brain dysfunction. Now, she would have a better chance of being called a neurologically impaired learning disabled child.

I met her quite by accident in a local business office. Since she is attractive and obviously bright, I enjoyed talking to her as I waited to see her employer. It didn't take long to learn that she was divorced twice, trying to support a child and about to be fired from her job. She was looking for another way to make a living. She is socially accomplished and asked pertinent questions about me and my work. She understood what I was saying and expressed concern about her seven-year-old who was having problems learning. She made a date to discuss it further.

When I began talking to her employer, I complimented him on having such a delightful person at the front desk. Sadly, he said they were going to terminate her in spite of her pleasant personality and willingness to try. Her clerical errors were beyond tolerance.

Not only did she make more than the usual letter reversals when typing, but she would leave out whole words or sentences. Words and sentences would be so mixed up that they made no sense even when the typing was straight copy work. When asked to correct errors, she was most pleasant, but she would then forget what was to be corrected and how. She might compound the errors in her attempt to correct them and might even include words that were not in the material at all.

When Marilyn came to my office about her child, we talked about brain dysfunction in more detail. Sometimes she would say, "That sounds like me."

I asked how well she had fared in school. The answer: "With extreme difficulty." She indicated that she'd always felt the need to stay very busy, so she had worked hard and somehow got by. As an aside, to our questions about some of her school activities, she told me that her parents had often teased her about being so clumsy that she bumped into walls.

After we talked some more, she asked if we would run an EEG on her. The results were abnormal. Some of the dysfunction was obviously genetic in nature, but some had apparently resulted from early injury. Since she was adopted and knew nothing about her natural parents, it was impossible to verify either.

Marilyn also took an IQ test. It showed her to be above average. She was not lacking in intelligence. She simply hadn't learned to read as others did. In addition, she had a problem with short-term memory loss. Her memory lapses alone made it hard for her to read with understanding. Even with remediation, she would never have been able to read well, but she could have done better with help. With some subject matter, she might have been taught by using recordings such as those made for the blind.

Now, Marilyn is trying to find something she can do well enough to support herself and her child. The search has been difficult. I learned recently that she has been discharged from several more secretarial positions and is now a "temporary" in a low level clerical job. This woman's story is a tragedy. The only fortunate thing is that her child can be helped.

I was greatly concerned recently when a local television station did a story on dyslexia. The implication of this particular report was that all dyslexia is hereditary. I don't believe that. In addition, the term dyslexia as it is used today is a catch-all for all reading disabilities. No two experts agree on a definition of the term itself. It follows, then, that such a blanket statement cannot be made. There are many types of reading problems and there are different sources for the disabilities.

My reasons for telling you Jane's and Marilyn's stories is that they both came into my circle accidentally, and as adults. Even Ray, who was referred to me by the court, was just short of being an adult. Herein lies my concern — that children will not be reached unless parents and teachers become aware that brain dysfunction does cause problems and that there are ways for experts to diagnose it. I know that the last thing any parent wants to hear is that something is wrong with Johnny's brain. But, if you are a practicing teacher, keep this information in mind. If you see certain signs or symptoms, in a particular child, ask your school's learning disability specialist or psychologist to visit your classroom. Ask them to observe what you've seen. They usually can find a tactful way to discuss the observations with the parents.

If you are a parent and observe a neighbor's child having problems, perhaps you can say, "Gee, I've just read an interesting book" and describe what's in it. Let's get these children the help that they need now so that as adults, they too can have a satisfactory life.

CHAPTER 3

MIRROR MIRROR ON THE WALL. . .

ANN called me about her son Jimmy when she heard from her friend about the kind of work we do. She was almost in tears as she said, "There's hardly anything in my house that isn't broken." When she sent Jimmy to his room as punishment for some of his behavior, instead of calming him down, it made him worse. He became so enraged, he just exploded—destroying his toys, tearing his clothes and the sheets on the bed, and even knocking holes in the wall—his room a shambles. She wanted to come and see us right then!

Early the next morning, Ann came to my office with Jimmy in tow. A five-and-one-half-year-old preschooler, the most noticeable thing upon meeting him is electric blond hair. It's the kind that stands on end no matter how much time or hair spray has been spent in the brushing of it. His eyes are wide set and his little fingers are curved but his overall appearance is attractive.

He hasn't been learning well in kindergarten even though recent formal testing by a psychologist gave an IQ score of 120, way above average. This is just one more problem on top of others for Ann and Jimmy. His behavior has been intolerable since he was three years old. He has had several professionals thoroughly puzzled

Jimmy could say words before he was eleven months old. At one year, he was putting several words together and assembling simple jigsaw puzzles. At two years old, he could do ten piece puzzles and could recite a children's book, "word for word." He was very active, even during sleep, but was a happy child.

18

However, since the age of three, Jimmy has been a severe discipline problem. His rages and tantrums can include kicking walls, messing his pants and smearing walls. It was at three than Ann first took him to a psychologist.

Within the past year or two, Jimmy has found it hard to comprehend or remember anything. He can only recognize five letters of the alphabet. He rarely sits down to do anything—like put a puzzle together—unless someone will sit down with him.

Jimmy either does nothing at all on his school papers or he does it all wrong. His teacher says he is easily distracted. She thinks he concentrates so much on trying to keep still, that he can't concentrate on what he is supposed to be doing. But, if he's not being still, he's a distraction to everyone else in the room. Ann noted that he had written his name backwards for the first few months of school.

Testing revealed that Jimmy had awkward, alternating hand movements which were more pronounced for the left hand. He could not stand for ten seconds on either foot, but again had more problems with the left. He yawned when he was asked to hyperventilate and also when he was stressed working on a test. His teacher had noticed that he often yawned a lot when she was trying to teach him, but she didn't think too much about it. A look in his mouth revealed a highly steepled palate (roof of mouth). He could not copy circles and squares. His circles looked like skinny eggs and his squares managed to have five sides. His EEG was abnormal.

Ann took the trouble to write up a family history. Neither Ann's husband nor daughter had any particular complaints or peculiarities for her to report. Nor was there anything in his family that indicated abnormalities might have been present.

However, Ann's brother had been "a handful." Ann told about a number of his escapades as a youngster. Their mother could never understand him. She also said that he has had trouble in his personal and business life as a result of his wild behavior. He still has a reading problem. Ann herself has had frequent headaches for years and still remembers how especially awful they were when she was taking tests in college. In addition, she sometimes had to be excused to run to the restroom because of stomach cramps, and as a kid she had had a lot of stomachaches.

Jimmy, her son, is fortunate that his brain dysfunction has been recognized, and at an early age. He won't be left to his own devices.

In his case, because of the nature of the EEG pattern, a trial on a medication was suggested *and* recommendations made to his teachers, and parents, of ways that they could go about teaching him more effectively in light of his learning deficits.

That was ten months ago. His "wild" and hyperactive behavior has been reduced. His next door neighbors didn't know that he had been tested, but they did notice how much more quietly he played in the backyard. And of course, his parents appreciate the calmer home atmosphere — no kicking walls in, etc. They are helping him every school day with his lessons and have set up a home program which will help him learn his letters and numbers.

I saw him three months ago, right before summer vacation. His EEG was much better. He didn't yawn when hyperventilating and was calmer. In fact, he sat for forty-five minutes drawing, while his parents and I talked. His interruptions were infrequent and he didn't wiggle or get up and down a lot.

His dad has accepted the possibility that Jimmy might not do too well in some subjects such as reading or arithmetic. But Jimmy is handling his body better and has good control of his large muscles. His father is talking about how good he is in sports and is encouraging him to develop these skills. Jimmy was in danger of being held back — another year in kindergarten. But now that his brain dysfunction has been diagnosed and he is getting the help he needs, he is entering the first grade and will have the opportunity to be a success, not a failure.

Sam, on the other hand, has more serious matters to deal with. He is eleven, the son of a former college athlete. His father is an engineer who had high hopes for his son both scholastically and athletically. The whole family will have to adjust to the idea that Sam will not fill their original expectations.

Sam, too, had been through learning and behavior problems when his parents brought him to us. A loner of long standing, he has been so frustrated by his poor reading skills that his mother reports, "He has cried his heart out." A number of his other skills test out at a seven or eight-year-old level. He is, to his advantage, a good listener. He has learned a great deal through listening and testing shows that he is not retarded.

Sam can't use his hands well. He has trouble standing or hopping on one foot at a time. These symptoms are more pronounced on the right side. He cannot handle his body well—he is clumsy. His dad had already noticed that Sam's concept of squares and triangles were out of the ordinary. His drawings were poorly defined. He has been in speech therapy for several years. Both of his little fingers are curved, his ears are low set, and the palate of his mouth is steepled. His EEG is abnormal and shows the kind of pattern not unusual in children with reading problems.

Sam can learn some coping skills and his social skills can be upgraded. His parents have located an excellent tutor to help with his learning disabilities, one who understands that Sam will never be able to do some things well. She has used the state services for the blind since he falls under the federal law covering neurological impairments. She has obtained educational tapes, and a machine on which to use them, even though there is nothing wrong with Sam's eyes.

Sam was placed in a learning disabled class where he can have some successes. A recent report says that he likes this new school. He is learning and gaining confidence as the weeks go by. Had he been seen earlier as Jimmy was, his academic and social life would have been much more enjoyable. And how much better might Marilyn have done had this sort of remediation been available to her?

In these last two cases, I've told you about certain physical features of these children. Now, it's time to tell you why certain minor physical irregularities or errors—called anomalies—which happen during fetal development *might* indicate irregularities in brain development also.

If physical irregularities are not too prominent or numerous, you can easily overlook them. Little Johnny may not be actually unattractive or obviously different. For instance, no face is exactly symmetrical. Johnny's is only a little more so than most kids—but not to the point of being disfigured. Only in such cases as Down's syndrome (mongoloids) will you see such an overwhelming degree of physical irregularities—downright deformities.

How and when do these developmental errors happen? It is believed they result from some kind of "insult" or unusual occurrence in the uterus during the first twelve or fourteen weeks of pregnancy. Toxic products in the mother's system, due to an illness, could be one cause. Another may be some genetic factor which produces toxicity during pregnancy. Males and females may react to this toxicity in different ways.

Sometimes investigations are done on animals to learn more about people. One such study on rats reported the effect of what happened during pregnancy and the behavior of the offspring after birth. On the eighth day of a twenty-one-day gestation, oxygen levels were lowered in the pregnant rats. These animals produced offspring which were hypo-emotional—they were underaroused and lethargic. This abnormal behavior persisted throughout the entire ninety days the animals were observed after birth. Monkeys subjected to reduced oxygen levels shortly after birth also had abnormal behaviors. They developed into animals which showed hyperactivity when first introduced into a new and unfamiliar situation. However, after they adapted to the situation they were hypo-emotional, as were the rats injured long before birth.

The brain develops along with other parts of the body, such as the face, arms and legs. The fingers, toes, eyes, ears and mouth are clearly defined at about the eighth week of pregnancy—well within the first trimester. Errors in development can occur for the head, face and extremities at this early stage. But the brain is also developing, and errors in its development may also be taking place at the same time. This is why anomalies in the parts of the body which are visible after birth may be important.

A relationship between minor physical anomalies and how some children do and act in school has been documented in quite a few studies. One study reported on a large number of first grade children examined for physical anomalies at the start of the school year. A list of common anomalies, such as given in Table I, were looked for in these children. The investigators used a weighting system as a way of handling and reporting the results. An anomaly with a weight or score of "two" indicated that the abnormality is either more important or more frequently seen than those with a "one." I have an artist sketch of what some of these anomalies look like (Fig. 3).

The children were grouped according to their total minor physical anomaly score. One group had no, or perhaps only one or two anomalies for a low anomaly score of "zero to three." None of these children appeared to have had any serious problems as they grew up. All behaved normally. All learned well enough to be promoted to the second grade.

The second group was made up of children with two and three

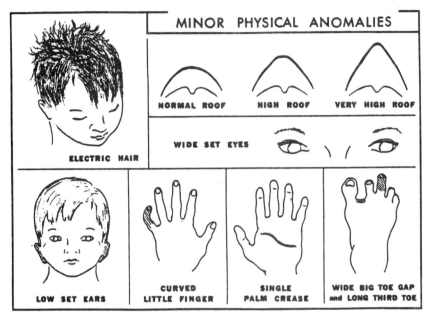

Figure 3.

minor abnormalities but with the anomaly score undr five. Of this group, 12 percent had to repeat the first grade.

The third group was comprised of children with the highest anomaly scores — over five. Sixty percent failed to be promoted to the second grade.

As infants, the children in this third group had in common a high degree of irritability. They tended to rock a lot, bang their heads and wake up frequently in the night. Allergies were also more common in these children.

In another study, infants were examined for physical anomalies within the first few days after birth, and were followed as they grew up. The children with the greater physical anomalies were more likely to show hyperactive behavior, some as early as two years old, than those with fewer anomalies. These children were less adaptable, less cooperative and more negative in manner. They were more apt to have short attention spans. Impulsiveness and aggression were fairly common. They were often described as excitable. They would overreact to unfavorable situations. They didn't seem to be as well motivated as those children with fewer or no anomalies.

Table I

COMMON MINOR PHYSICAL ANOMALIES

Visible Sign	Weight Score
_____ HEAD _____	
"Electric hair"	
fine hair that won't comb down	2
fine hair that is soon awry after combing	1
_____ EYES _____	
Wide set eyes	
approximate distance between tear ducts:	
greater than 1.5 inches	2
1.25-1.5 inches	1
_____ EARS _____	
Low set	
bottom of ears in line with:	
mouth (or lower)	2
between mouth and nose	1
No "free" ear lobes (lobes attached to head)	2
_____ MOUTH _____	
High palate	
roof of mouth:	
highly steepled	2
moderately high (flat and narrow at top)	1
_____ HANDS _____	
Little finger	
markedly curved toward other fingers	2
slighly curved toward other fingers	1
One crease across the palm instead of two	1
_____ FEET _____	
Third toe	
definitely longer than second toe	2
equal in length to second toe	1
Wide gap, 1.25 inch or more, between big and second toe	1
Webbing between second and third toes	1

Once the unusual behavior began, *it didn't go away*.

A higher percentage of boys had problems. This, in itself, is not remarkable. You may already know that many more boys are conceived than girls. Many more males are miscarried or stillborn. Of the surviving males, a higher percentage succumb to crib deaths and other childhood illnesses. Continuing on into adulthood, males are more likely to experience stress-related ailments and, in fact, die from them. It's certainly no secret that there are many more elderly women than men.

This is not to say that girls shouldn't be carefully observed for that combination of symptoms that indicate a possible brain dysfunction. As you've seen with Jane and Marilyn, they are now disadvantaged adults because their difficulties went unnoticed.

Remember the old nursery rhyme:

> What are little girls made of?
> Sugar and spice and everything nice.
> What are little boys made of?
> Snips and snails and puppy dog tails.

This is a bit of joking wisdom made many years before science could prove the less obvious differences between the sexes. While many of the girls were hyperactive, often it was not to the same degree. They were more likely to be overly "busy." Actually, a higher percentage of the girls were hypoactive; that is, they were shy, inactive, repeated actions or thoughts in an automatic way — as opposed to easily adopting new procedures and they didn't make friends with other children easily.

Of course, some of the differences in behavior between boys and girls may have to do with social conditioning. After all, people tend to expect and tolerate a "Peck's bad boy." Girls are supposed to be "good." It's also believed by some that hormonal differences between the sexes can have some effect on behavior. Others think the mother's own hormonal system may have a different effect on a male and female fetus.

Dr. Kent Durfee has identified what he calls "crooked ears and the bad boy syndrome." This can be easily checked by placing your index fingers in each of the child's ear canals. Visualize a line running from one finger to the other through the head. Dr. Durfee found that fifteen out of seventeen boys whose *ear canals* were *uneven* did poorly on visual-motor perception tests. They had difficulty processing sensory information. They showed a wide range of other problems including poor handwriting, spelling and reading. He and

I agree that early diagnosis of brain dysfunction is essential. He, too, insists that taking a chance on "waiting for the child to outgrow it" is asking for profound problems later.

Another area of concern that may relate to brain dysfunction is child abuse. The study of infant anomalies also reported that mothers of children with numerous minor physical abnormalities appeared to be less supportive of their children. It would appear that those mothers reacted to the children, not necesarily the other way around. The mothers seemed to be more restrictive than those mothers of children with no or few abnormalities. There appeared to be a circular interaction between parent and child and often the child was physically abused.

Little Johnny, by virtue of a central nervous system impairment, may have been excessively demanding and disruptive when his requests were not met immediately. Mother, in turn became more restrictive or used punishment. Angry, Johnny then punished Mother with hostility. The chain perpetuated itself with still further reactions and/or punishment.

There was no way either Johnny or Mother could know there was a reason for his irritable behavior. They were simply locked in a battle from the start. To make matters worse, it was possible that Johnny could have inherited some of his traits from Mother. It could well have been that neither had good emotional control. In any case, their poor relationship could have been caused, a least in part, by the congenital or birth characteristics of the child rather than by the mother's inability to parent properly.

This idea is further backed up by observations of social workers whose jobs require them to place children in foster homes. They have found that there are some children who cannot be placed anywhere with success. These children get shuttled from one foster home to another because even the best of foster parents cannot put up with them. Where some of these children are concerned, social workers have found it virtually impossible to find a compatible foster parent.

Mind you, I'm not trying to relieve parents of the responsibility for child abuse, but these reports do make you wonder if it would be profitable to test the children in such cases. In how many cases could the child's brain dysfunction be the underlying cause? We don't know, but it could be worth investigating.

CHAPTER 4

NOW YOU SEE THEM, NOW YOU DON'T

A LMOST all of us have had a routine physical examination in a
doctor's office. One of the things he did was to check out reflexes. He tapped below your knee with a little rubber hammer and
your leg flew up — or I hope it did. This response or "kick" is called a
hard neurological sign. Most of the hard signs are reflex responses,
and they give an indication of the condition of our central nervous
system. Unless there is an injury or some kinds of illness, the kick
and other reflexes will be present from infancy.

The soft signs, however, evolve and become more evident as a
child matures. They are non-reflex in nature, but they are still sensitive indicators of central nervous system dysfunction. Many are
based on what the child should be able to do at a given age. Usually,
normal is judged according to the age of the child. You wouldn't expect a child of two to perform some tasks as well as a child of seven.
Yet, when a seven-year-old can perform no better than a four-year-
old, there may be trouble. A parent or teacher can learn about many
of these "soft signs" without formal training.

One group of soft signs has to do with the inability to coordinate
the large muscles of the body properly. As we grow and develop, our
ability to make our muscles work together increases. It's a matter of
what the child should be able to do at a given age.

You already know that Johnny cannot begin to stand on one foot
when he is two years old. He will certainly fall. But, if he cannot do
this well at age seven without losing his balance, and if he still can't
do this one year later, it may be one indicator of brain dysfunction.

Perhaps you will remember a segment of "60 Minutes" that aired on January 16, 1983. It told of the tragic life led by a young man, an epileptic, not convulsive, who had been misdiagnosed as paranoid schizophrenic. After many horrible and inexcusable incidents had happened to him, he made contact with a doctor at Harvard who determined what the real problem was. As his story unfolded, it was evident that many things had been overlooked when he was a child.

First, he was a school dropout when he joined the Marines at seventeen years old. While no details were given, the implication was that he had had school problems or he would not hve dropped out. His speech was somewhat "mushy," a soft neurological sign. The doctor also did some testing and discovered that he couldn't do such a simple thing as to walk backwards with his eyes closed, another soft neurological sign.

We know of other cases where young men have been discharged from the service because they could not stand at attention. It was, for them, a physical impossibility — a brain-related disability.

We need to make the differentiation between *gross* and *fine* motor control, too. Let's relate it to the cases we've already talked about.

Ray had sufficient gross motor control to play football fairly well, but his fine motor control left something to be desired. When writing and drawing, he couldn't connect lines with other lines. Pencil pressure would vary greatly, sometimes the paper would be torn by excessive pressure. His hand work was, in a word, sloppy.

Jane, on the other hand, had good handwriting and could draw well, but she tended to stagger when walking. She was inclined to fall, especially going up and down stairs. Marilyn was also clumsy. Sam will never be the athlete his father hoped for. They had problems with gross motor control. In Jane's case, this lack of control was apparently genetic since she reported that her mother did the same thing.

The Thompson family presented us with an opportunity to run EEGs on three members of the family. You have already been shown these EEGs in Figure 1. They are a good example of brain dysfunction that is genetic in origin. Two of them also appear to have an additional or "acquired" dysfunction.

Our initial contact with them was through Butch, a high school football player. He was referred because he had developed chronic headaches and insomnia and they thought that he might have had a head injury while playing football. He had "blacked out" once on the football field.

Mrs. Thompson described Butch as always having been extremely active and accident prone. He had suffered many skinned knees and broken bones. Yet, with the exception of the headaches, Butch rarely seemed to feel pain.

Scholastically, his achievements could be described as uneven. His grades would fluctuate widely. His family thought that this was because he was only doing his homework half-heartedly at times. He has been a nail biter since infancy. During testing, he couldn't stand on his right leg without losing his balance; he could accomplish this on his left leg. He laughs nervously and inappropriately. His parents told me that he was always "fidgety" and that it was hard for him to calm down after coming in from school or football practice.

As we asked about the rest of the family, it came out that the father, Steve, had experienced chronic headaches since childhood. He had a hard time learning in school. Although he didn't complain of serious insomnia, he didn't sleep well either. Steve knew he was "not as smart" as his brothers or his wife, but he accepted this. He sometimes has episodes of uncontrollable anger, but he is not violent. He, too, has a balance problem. He is one of those young men who was discharged from the service because he couldn't stand at attention without weaving about. He was so poor at sports when he was a child that he would not participate.

Carol, a younger daughter, has been hyperactive since birth. Like Steve, she has a relatively "short fuse," but not to the point of attacking or destroying anything. She can watch television longer at a time than can Butch. She, too, has a learning disability and as with Butch and Steve, she was unsuccessful at balancing on her right leg. During testing, she showed excessive twitching which, under pressure, became jerky.

These three members of the family did not have identical symptoms, but the similarities are enough to indicate that heredity did play its part. As you look at their EEG tracings, the patterns look pretty much alike for Butch, Steve and Carol. Neither the mother nor the other son had similar problems.

Let's look over the symptoms again: a balance problem, chronic headaches, flashes of temper, sleeping problems, inability to feel pain normally, nervous laughter, excessive twitching and short attention span. Some medication was suggested for Butch *and* his difficulty was explained to him in a way that he could accept. Now, one-and-one-half years later, he is less fidgety and is having an easier time of it. Of course, there are the usual problems and anxieties that go along with being a junior in high school. Carol is in a learning disabilities class for some subjects. We are following her also. Steve likes his new "behind the scenes" job with the same company — less stress — and he is enjoying a hobby he always wanted — woodworking and overall first-class "fix-it" person.

Since nature has endowed the average school child with a grace of movement that is a pleasure to watch, their clumsiness should have been noticed. Amidst the beauty of most children's movements, it is hard to miss the child who falls over his own feet, has difficulty keeping his balance and knocks over the potted plant on the teacher's desk. Their clumsiness is more than just poor muscle movement. Some of these children *lack* the *ability* to build up patterns of movements that form the basis of smooth performance. At first glance, it's not unusual for many such children to be considered as having low intellectual ability. But, remember, I've said before that their IQs can range from normal to gifted. We know of one very clumsy but gifted boy who wants to be a chemist. He will make an outstanding theorist, but it would be a disaster to let him handle the equipment. He will need assistants to carry out the delicate work of the laboratory. But he will be able to cope *if* the clumsiness is taken into account.

What follows are some simple little soft sign tests. A child's inability to carry them out successfully will NOT tell you he or she needs to be tested for brain dysfunction. The results will only tell you that one individual, particularly in the first or second grade, is not keeping up with the average child in these abilities.

Teachers may choose to have a class do some of these exercises together. This way, no one should feel singled out. You may find that there are several clumsy children in the room. Even at the first grade level, if a child has learning and behavior problems and some gross muscle incoordination, you may want to look for other physical clues.

I have described many of these tests in some detail, including the score needed to pass. I hope that parents and teachers will use them. They can be played like a game. Don't let the words "test" and "pass" scare you. These tests or abilities are but one indication that a child might need to be seen and tested by a professional.

Motor impersistence is the inability to maintain, that is persist in, certain acts for even brief periods of time.

1. Ask the child to stand still, eyes closed and feet together, head upright and arms outstretched, fingers of both hands extended and separated. He should be able to hold this position for ten to fifteen seconds without shuffling the feet, moving the body, or opening the eyes. Under six, children often need a few movements of the ankles and toes to maintain balance. You can expect optimal performance for those over seven. At this point, you watch for twitching movements in the arms, fingers, neck and trunk. You may also see a swaying of the body.

2. Have the child stick out his tongue as far as possible. Two five-second trials are given. Withdrawal of the tongue before the time is up constitutes failure.

3. Ask the child to take a deep breath and say "ah" as long as he can. Again, two trials are allowed. A combined total of eighteen or more seconds is normal. Each trial should last at least seven seconds.

There are many forms of testing for motor control. Here are a few:

4. Probably the simplest "test" in the world is to hand a child a paper clip and three or four pieces of paper. Such an exercise actually requires complex integration of actions. The child is asked to "clip them together neatly as fast as you can." He or she is observed for clumsiness, not supporting the paper near the clip and even for not knowing which end of the paper clip to use. Important is to watch for uncontrolled movements of other muscle groups called "associated movements" and "motor overflow." Examples are readily apparent in the mouth or face such as wrinkling the forehead, grimacing, screwing up the side of the mouth and licking the lips. Another form is seen in some children who make similar muscle movements with the opposite hand (mirror movements) while they work. Children of six or seven should not have many of these movements.

5. Most children can rapidly touch each finger, in order, with their thumbs and then reverse the order. Done with each hand, this shows up awkwardness in fine muscle movements of the fingers.

The test is demonstrated with a "Watch me first." Then a "Now you do it—now a little faster—now the other hand." The examiner looks for inability to curl fingers, missed contacts, poor sequence, slowness, "stickiness" of release and reckless speed with inaccuracy. Slight mirror movements in the fingers of the other hand has been reported to be normal up to about age eleven. If a child cannot do this and has had trouble with other tests, this is an additional clue to possible brain dysfunction.

6. One particularly sensitive test of motor control is the ability to perform rapidly alternating or reversing movements. A child and the examiner sit in chairs facing each other. The examiner places his hand on his knee, palm down, and shows the child very slowly how to slap his knee alternately with his palm and then the back of his hand. The child is asked to do the same thing. At first he is told to "go slow," then "faster," then "very fast." The child's wrists and arms must be lifted—not allowed to rest against the thigh. Each hand is tested separately and then both hands together. Some children are unable to maintain this reversing pattern of motion. After a few alternations, they just pat the thigh with the palms of their hands. Others cannot maintain a smooth performance. They break the pattern and pick it up again. Still others have awkward or slow movements. It may be a child can do the pattern well with one hand and not the other. This would suggest that the opposite side of the brain is more dysfunctioned. At six or seven years of age, children are still likely to be a little awkward. Pauses may occur at the point of reversing the hand, i.e., "sticky turns." At eight, however, the motion should be quite smooth.

Tests of finger localization can be valuable in looking for possible brain dysfunction. The inability to recognize which fingers are being touched with eyes closed is called "finger agnosia." Actually, in the "touch" exercises illustrated for you in Figure 4 two abilities are involved: simple touch-recognition and a form of perceptual-spatial ability.

7. In the finger differentiation test, the child places his hand on the table and stretches it out. While the child watches, he is shown how sometimes two points on the same finger will be touched at the same time and sometimes just one point on two fingers next to each other. In the test proper, the child closes his eyes and is

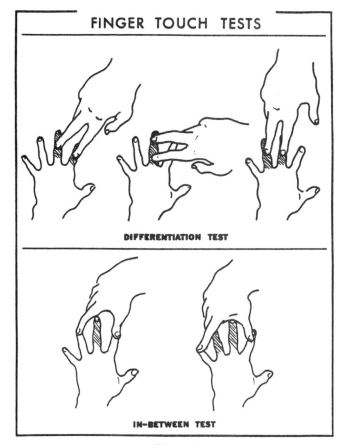

FINGER TOUCH TESTS

DIFFERENTIATION TEST

IN-BETWEEN TEST

Figure. 4

asked, "How many fingers am I touching — one or two?" The examiner maintains contact until an answer is given. The child is permitted to open his eyes to verify his answer. This procedure is repeated eight times, four trials on each hand. Two trials touching the same finger and two touching adjacent fingers are given in irregular sequence. Six correct answers are considered a "pass." Most children can pass this test by age seven and a half.

8. In the "in-between" test, which is the one with the spatial element, two of the child's fingers are touched at the same time. The examiner asks, "How many fingers are there in-between the ones I'm touching — how many in the middle? Now there are two in the middle — now there is one — now there aren't any." After the

child understands what it is he has to do, he closes his eyes and the test begins. Finger contact is maintained until the child answers. Then he can open his eyes to see if his answer was correct. The test is repeated four times on each hand. The finger pairs are touched in irregular sequence covering the pair combinations: once with no fingers in-between, twice with one finger, and once with two fingers in-between. Six correct answers out of eight are a "pass." Children of eight pass this test.

There appears to be a rather strong relationship between some types of reading problems and finger agnosia. Some even regard finger agnosia as a good indicator of future reading problems. Some children with finger agnosia rotate letters. Some may have a spelling problem. Errors usually involve the inability to properly serialize letters in a word whether written or spelled aloud. Slow readers may also have such a serializing deficit in addition to their other reading problems.

Children who fail "finger tests" may fail right-left discrimination tests as well. Some children with finger agnosia have difficulty speaking clearly. It will show up when asked to say such a nonsense phrase as "puh-tuh-kuh" rapidly for five seconds.

Children with reading and writing problems may have difficulty copying simple designs. This same difficulty is also seen in adults after certain types of strokes. Children's drawings are an easy way to get many important clues as to what is going on with them. We use a certain set of designs — the Bender Gestalt test — and ask the child to copy them.

Drawings are something that people can easily understand. So to build up to my point of how revealing drawings can be, I will show you how some adults and children did this test (Figs. 5–8). The first test in Figure 5 shows the designs in this drawing test and how they are normally drawn — with some reasonable variation. What a diffrence in the drawings on the right! They were made by a person who had a stroke two and one-half years before. Note the heavy pressure on the pencil, the reversing of designs, the shaky lines which indicates his fine hand tremor, and so forth.

The next drawings show how operating on the deep brain can affect one's visual peception (Fig. 6). This man had Parkinson's disease — shaking palsy. He had surgery done to relieve his tremor. His drawings on the left, done before surgery, were not too large to

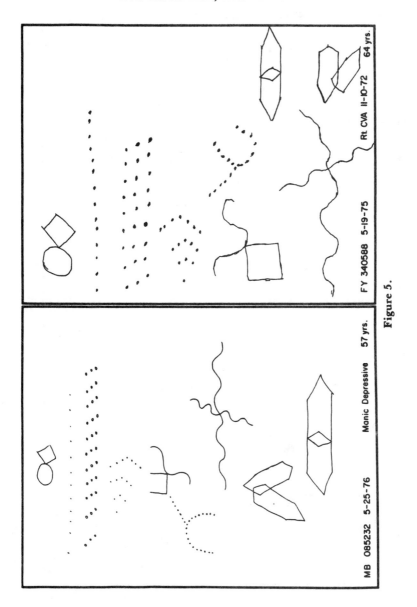

Figure 5.

start with. After the surgery, they were practically microscopic. This demonstrates beautifully how the lowly deep brain affects our behavior—in this case our visual-perceptual ability.

The drawings in Figure 7 were done by a sixteen-year-old girl

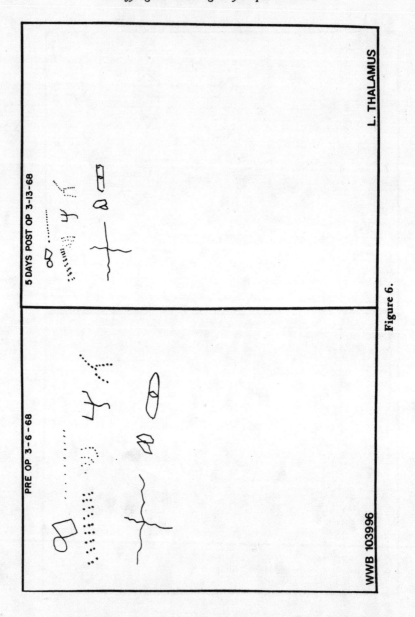

Figure 6.

who had finally been sent for evaluation. All of this time, it was thought that she was not too bright, even mentally retarded. She was a nice, friendly and social girl. Her reading ability was only primary school level. Her spelling was terrible. But she appeared sharp! Her intelligence test scores proved our impression right—scores in the middle average range—far from retarded. She is, and always has been, a neurologically impaired learning-disabled student—one with a severe reading impairment. Her EEG was abnormal. See how she drew the designs in the test. It is obvious to almost everyone that one of her problems is a visual-perceptual deficit. Too bad she is now sixteen! How much brighter her future would have been had this testing been done preschool.

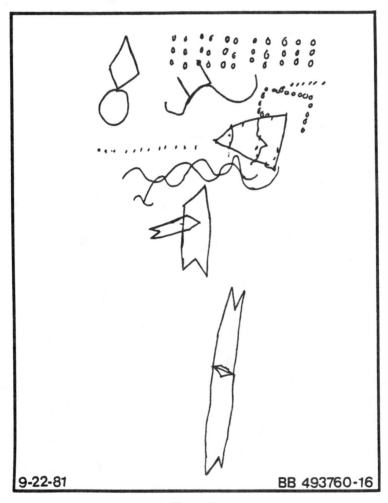

9-22-81   BB 493760-16

Figure 7.

We have the drawings of two younger children, nine-and-one-half and eleven-and-one-half-years old, to show you (Fig. 8). Both of them were sent by the school system, both had learning disabilities and one was hyperactive. An abnormal EEG was found in both. Note the small drawings and how they are crowded at the top of the page. There are also figure reversals and other perception problems. The student who drew the designs on the right could not do angles at age eleven-and-one half.

To summarize — what do we look for in drawings? Corners that don't meet and lines that overextend. Heavy pencil pressure — sometimes almost tearing the paper. The size of the drawings . . . are they roughly the size presented, or are they extremely small or extremely large? Do the drawings overlap or bump into each other? How are they placed on the paper? Are they spaced rather well or are they up at the top of the page, near the bottom, or at the very sides of the page?

I have also illustrated a little drawing exercise that you can give a young child (Fig. 9). The child is asked to copy a circle, triangle, square, rectangle and diamond. Note how, and if, he closes his designs and how he executes angles. For example, does the triangle look like an Indian tepee and does the diamond have "ears"? "Ears" occur because the child has misjudged the direction needed to close the diamond and he tries to correct or compensate for the error.

These figures are considered within the skill range of the pre-primary child. Children normally should be able to draw them successfully at six years of age. The diamond design may take a year longer.

Besides the drawings themselves, watch how the child handles the paper. Is the paper placed at an unusual angle? Does the child turn the paper instead of moving the pencil? For example, does he turn the paper to draw a square so that the figure is completed by a single motion of the hand instead of lifting the pencil up from the paper to form the sides? Some authorities believe that these simple form-copying tests can predict arithmetic skill and reading success or failure.

These apparent eccentricities are not indications that the child needs glasses. Nothing is wrong with his eyes. He is recreating the drawings — the way he actually perceives and can do them.

If Johnny consistently presents you with original drawings

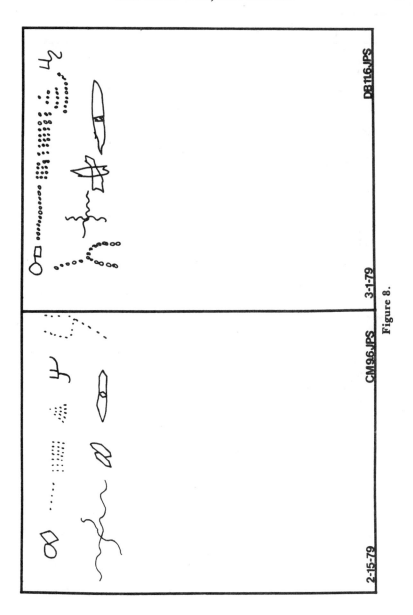

Figure 8.

placed at the top, left-hand portion of his paper, store that information away while you check for other things. Is his handwriting extremely small? Is the pencil pressure inconsistent? These are a few

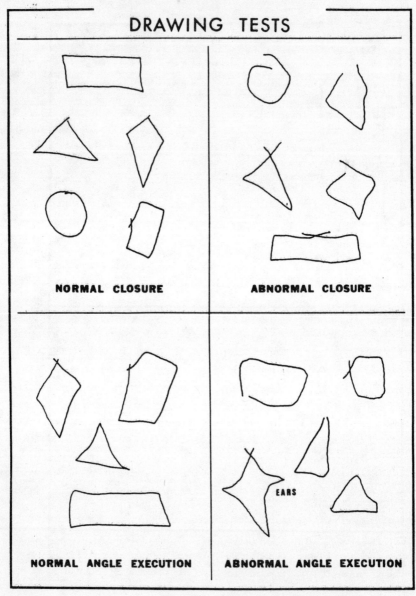

DRAWING TESTS

NORMAL CLOSURE

ABNORMAL CLOSURE

NORMAL ANGLE EXECUTION

ABNORMAL ANGLE EXECUTION

EARS

Figure 9.

simple things you can look for in a classroom setting or at home with your child. Please do so—the child you help may be your own.

CHAPTER 5

THAT'S STRANGE BEHAVIOR!

THERE are brain-based symptoms that are often ignored or diagnosed as something else. One group can appear in the form of chronic stomachaches or gastrointestinal disturbances. Children having unaccounted for stomachaches may show EEG patterns of the same type seen in patients who have seizures. These stomachaches are not seizures as we know them, but the abnormal brain wave activity is similar. These cases have what is called an *epileptiform* or an *epileptic equivalent* symptom.

Since the brain controls or mediates the movements of the smooth muscles of the stomach and intestine, it can cause abnormal functioning of this system. Stomachaches can appear spontaneously when the child is under some kind of stress. Sometimes, the pain is localized and can be mistaken for appendicitis.

Certain types of chronic headaches are associated with an abnormal EEG. These headaches seem to defy explanation and sometimes have been dismissed as tension headaches. Most of the time they are generalized, although some are localized. Nausea, vomiting and dizziness can accompany the headaches. Again, if these symptoms appear in combination with others, such as soft neurological signs, learning deficits and behavior problems, they are worth adding to the list of indicators of possible brain dysfunction.

Yawning, in the extreme, is another physical clue. Normally, it simply reflects fatigue or boredom. Teachers will put up with yawning unless it is too flagrant; then they view yawning as a sign of boredom or disrespect. They certainly rarely interpret it as an abnormal bit of behavior even when it is excessive.

Nevertheless, the child who yawns excessively is usually under some kind of stress. We see it in its most pronounced form in children who have been referred to us for behavior and learning disorders. Most of the time, the yawning has not been reported as part of the total picture. But we've had at least one child whose yawning was so frequent that it actually interfered with the testing itself. This child had a highly abnormal EEG. Usually, we see the yawning symptom appear as we ask the patient to hyperventilate for a few minutes. We ask him to breathe deeply to create a kind of stress while we are running the EEG.

Sometimes adult patients, who have had deep brain surgery for Parkinson's disease, will yawn just like the children with a brain dysfunction. This may continue for several months after surgery. This leads us to believe that the deep brain is involved with this type of behavior in children. When these brain structures are disturbed, yawning occurs in situations that would not ordinarily trigger it.

Some researchers think excessive yawning may be a sign of a less developed brain. They equate this with the prominent yawning of baboons under stress. For a baboon, this is stereotyped behavior; but we see it happen in higher primates such as young rhesus monkeys when they are stressed. The tendency is, therefore, to believe that excessive yawning in children could be an indication of a developmental deficit. It's certainly a response researchers continue to observe closely.

Allergies and asthmatic attacks have been the subject of recent studies in connection with brain dysfunction. Asthma attacks may well reduce the amount of oxygen necessary to proper brain functioning and, in time, do some harm. On the other hand, one study suggests that some allergies may be caused by pre-existing brain dysfunction. If a child who has some of the other indicators or problems, and also has allergies and/or asthma, these can be added to your list and can be a deciding reason for taking the child for testing.

We are still researching the functions of the deep brain as it may be involved in the excessive motion of a hyperactive child or the nervous laughter or giggles of another child — the type of laughter that may make him stand out from all others in a classroom. When stressed, as during a work assignment, this child smiles in a shallow manner and giggles. The response is inappropriate for the situation.

The child may also be restless or impulsive in other situations. Actually, this particular form of giggling and smiling is involuntary—in some children, even epileptiform behavior.

Nervous laughter may be a relative of a form of seizure which appears in a rare form of epilepsy: *gelastic* epilepsy or laughing fits. Explosive hyperactive behavior may be related to another rare form of epilepsy: *cursive* epilepsy or running fits. In neither type of epilepsy does the person display convulsive movements. In the first there is the uncontrollable mirthless laughter; in the other the person explodes into compulsive uncontrollable running. In both cases, the abnormal electrical activity appears to affect a single behavior in a limited way.

While it is true that these forms of epilepsy are rare, it is now thought that a milder version of the same behaviors, the laughter and "running fits" may represent fragments of a seizure pattern— another clue that something may be wrong.

Today, you may be told that a child has epilepsy, but you seldom see a seizure because very good medication has been developed to keep it under control. The most easily recognized type involves convulsive movements. These convulsions represent the electrical activity of the brain really going "haywire." It is impossible to ignore someone having this type of *grand mal* or *major motor* seizure. The older term grand mal is derived from the French and Latin to convey the meaning of a spectacular event. The *mal* from "malum" meaning "ill" is combined with the word *grand* "large" to mean large illness.

Seizures can be caused by abnormal electrical activity in the whole brain or in just a certain area of the brain. Seizures, such as the violent and disturbed type that the young man interviewed by "60 MINUTES" had, may begin in an area of the brain called the temporal lobe. Often, the only thing the person remembers is the initial anger.

It is important to know that a "true" seizure is rarely aggressive. Could a person during a seizure pull out a gun and shoot someone? The answer is hardly. These persons may swear, spit and show hostility during a seizure, but they are much too confused to carry out any *organized* illegal activity. Studies have shown that they only try to go on the defensive when threatened or someone attempts to restrain them. If aggression is present, it is so disorganized and stereotyped and not of the type likely to be associated with well-directed and premeditated criminal behavior.

Sometimes, when we run an EEG, we get dramatic happenings that makes a wonderful illustration — a seizure that didn't appear to be a seizure. This is the story, with accompanying EEG, of a boy who was a destructive fifteen-year-old adolescent who had a behavior problem with a learning disability. His early history reads: . . . five weeks premature, had to be resuscitated, first convulsion age nine months, three more during infancy, then none until four years of age. . . . Temper tantrums started at age two. . . . "diagnosed" as a hyperactive child at age four . . . destructive at home, hard to manage . . . would get up on a cabinet, empty it out, throw out flour, sugar, etc. . . when finished drinking, he would throw his glasses in the sink and break them.

Now, to the EEG drama as it unfolds in Figure 10. While he was hyperventilating (a standard procedure in the test), this teenager began to smile and look around as is noted on the actual EEG tracing. Follow the events in the upper half of the illustration: he smiles, yawns, restless movements . . . stretches and smiles. Then, in the lower half of the illustration, the patient stops hyperventilating . . . seizure activity! See the big slow waves . . . and the notation: patient smiles during this discharge of seizure activity. There was no shaking, no drooling at the mouth, etc. If you had asked him a question or told him something during this discharge, he more than likely would not remember it later.

How does he behave now as an adolescent? He hits both parents, likes to play with younger children and bullies them, likes to fight. It is important to note that there are times when he will strike or bite someone and not be aware of what he is doing. He has a school history of hyperactivity, and teachers have never wanted him in their classes. Until last year, he was in a learning disability class. He gets A's in reading and writing, F's in math and science. So, not all children with brain dysfunction have reading problems, some have trouble in other subjects.

There are several important physical facts about the boy: he drinks fluids excessively (may even get up at night, go to the kitchen, and drink a gallon or more of water); he has unusual temperature tolerances (in cold weather he goes out in the yard without any shoes and only a T-shirt on and says he's warm; in the summer he wears the normal amount of clothing and says that "it

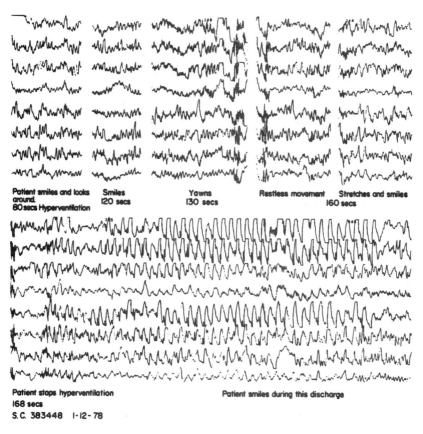

Figure 10.

seems as if he is turned around"); he has a restricted sweating pattern (has been noted to perspire in his scalp and eyebrows but not on his face and neck); and now he is having headaches daily. One of the patient's diagnoses is psychomotor seizures.

There are "small illness" seizures (sometimes called petit mal) and these are the ones that are least likely to be noticed unless you know what you're looking for. They often are in the form of "absences" or little periods of unawareness. There is no muscle movement. There is just a momentary break in the stream of thought or activity. These episodes are referred to as *epileptic absences* or *simple absence seizures*. In some small seizures there may be blinking of the eyes or minor twitchings of the eyelids and muscles around the eyes.

There may be barely visible movements of muscles in the hands and arms. These forms of seizures with such muscle movements make up the grouping *minor motor epilepsy*.

Sometimes, a child will be scolded, unjustifiably, by the teacher or parent because he appears not to pay attention. Yet, a seizure disorder can be the reason for a child seeming to lose the continuity of school work. If a number of these absences occur in a thirty-minute period, the child is missing a good bit of classroom work.

The term "true petit mal" is usually reserved for a type of seizure which has a very *specific* form of seizure activity in the EEG. This is called the "petit mal" wave. The blinking of the eyes which may accompany this kind of epilepsy is synchronized with, and occurs at the same three per second rate, as the petit mal seizure waves in the EEG. This fine distinction in wave forms is important in this instance, because "true" petit mal epilepsy requires a specific type of anticonvulsant medication.

There are odd forms of behavior in epilepsy. A young woman we saw had *complex partial epilepsy* known in the older terminology as *psychomotor epilepsy*. This is taken from the Greek *psyche*, meaning "soul," principle of life or mind, and *motor* from the Latin "motus" to move. Persons with this form of epilepsy may perform a series of coordinated acts that are out of place, even bizarre. They serve no useful purpose and are not remembered later.

This woman removed all the dishes from the kitchen cupboard and then immediately and methodically replaced them but could not remember doing this. Witnesses thought it amusing. After they told her what she had done, she laughed as if it were a funny story. "I was so tired, I must have been asleep on my feet," she commented.

But, at thirty she had an illness that began with a convulsion. It was followed by a high fever. The convulsion was interpreted as being part of the illness. About a year later, however, she had an "unprovoked" seizure while attending a movie. She woke up in a hospital. The diagnosis was finally made: epilepsy. She had experienced not one but two grand mal seizures.

Other people with this form of epilepsy, complex partial epilepsy, may seem preoccupied and have a peculiar mannerism. You might see a man stroking his hair or simply rolling the thumb against his fingers. Another may appear to be picking lint from her clothes. You yourself probably know someone with a habit that you thought was odd or have observed a stranger doing something "weird." Some of these people may be actually having a form of seizure. Petit mal and absence seizures, on the other hand, may be interpreted as "taking a minute to think" or being "at a loss for words," or "having a nervous tic." Sometimes, when occurring repeatedly over a long period of time, the child may be considered emotionally disturbed. "Johnny just retreats into his own little world."

I have given you information about different forms of seizures, not to frighten you but to show you that there *may* be a relationship between little Johnny staring off into space and a possible brain dysfunction. You cannot diagnose any form of epilepsy in the classroom or at home any more than you can diagnose brain dysfunction itself. Both require neurological testing. But the symptoms I've talked about in Chapters 3, 4, and 5 can indicate that testing would be advisable. If you child has some of these symptoms and you think that "something" is wrong, you have nothing to lose by taking him in for testing.

CHAPTER 6

WHAT GOES ON IN THE HEAD OFFICE?
OR WHAT'S A BRAIN FOR?

IN a sense, we have two brains—an old brain and a new brain. In lower animals the *ratio* of new brain to old brain is significantly less than in human beings. For example, in a primitive group of animals, the insectivores, which include such animals as the tree shrew and hedgehog, there is little new brain relative to old brain. As animals advance in the evolutionary scale, the *ratio* of new brain to old brain increases.

The old brain is located below the new brain and is often called the deep brain. Other terms used are lower brain primitive brain, and subcortical brain. It is that part of our brain most similar to that of other animals. Although the old brain or deep brain may be "primitive," it is a very important part of our whole brain. It receives stimuli or messages from our eyes, ears, arms, legs, and even our internal organs, such as the stomach, and sends these messages to the new brain. The new brain cannot function well if the old or deep brain does not function well. The deep brain is selective in what it sends up to the new brain, allowing some stimuli to pass and not transmitting other stimuli.

A person's deep brain might be unable to sift stimuli properly which could result in a low tolerance for stress. It does not matter if the stress is physical or emotional, some individuals always need a "lead time." Surprises upset them and they may "black out" if too much is happening. When bombarded with too much information at one time, whether in a social or learning situation, they become con-

48

fused. Their new or upper brain is simply not getting the appropriate information on which to act—it's getting way too much. These people tend to withdraw from stressful situations and often "fly off the handle" if they can't. They fare better in more structured situations.

On the other hand, some persons may need more stimulation than they are getting. The lower brain may not be sending sufficient stimuli to the upper brain. These are our "always on the go" people. They may be underaroused and race around looking for something more.

Our "gray matter," which most of us consider the brain (not true), is part of our new brain or upper brain. This matter is the cortex or cortical tissue, and together with the "white matter," the axons or nerve fibers, which are projections of the cortical cells, make up the new brain. In the development of the brain, the new brain is formed around "hollows," or sacs, called the ventricles. The ventricles contain the cerebrospinal fluid which nourishes and "bathes" the brain. In this fluid, besides the brain sugar, there are the neurotransmitters and other brain chemicals which transmit the electrical signals the brain generates from the sugar it uses. One form of these signals we record as an EEG.

We develop a very refined cortex which is divided into four major areas or lobes for each side of the brain: the frontal, parietal, occipital and temporal lobes. The occipital lobes are our visual analyzer. The parietal lobes, among its other functions, enable us to operate in the visual-spatial areas needed for reading and writing. Also, they "recognize" and make us aware of such stimuli as pain, temperature, touch, pressure and muscle position. They even enable us to locate ourselves geographically in space.

The temporal lobes control our speech, articulation, word fluency and memory abilities. Areas in this lobe which process auditory stimuli make us aware of sounds and what kind of sounds; in other words, our hearing analyst. In addition to all of that, certain of the temporal lobe structures are a kind of policeman. They police our aggressive behavior (our anger, rages and temper tantrums) and try to keep our behavior within acceptable limits. The temporal lobe the "youngest" member of our brain: it is the last added in the evolutionary process and it is the first to age. The frontal lobes, especially wonderful in the human being, allow us to "think"—that is, to work in the abstract, to plan, to decide, and even to change our minds in mid-course if necessary.

None of the lobes of the brain operate entirely independently. They must function together, sending messages back and forth through an intricate wiring system. Indeed, there are even more parts of the brain system in between the deep brain and the gray matter, all of which are important to the proper functioning of all the other parts. Difficulties in any portion of the brain can affect either behavior or learning ability, or both. If memory cannot be stored properly, learning is extremely difficult. If there is little control exercised by the upper brain—either through damage to its lobes or a faulty transmission network—behavior can be less than perfect.

To give you some knowledge about the operation of the brain, I will compare the brain with a large business operation. All of us have had some experience with those. We are aware that there are many electrical lines and many telephone lines in any building of great size. There are also the plumbing and heating pipes. The building would be useless without them. These necessary items might be compared with the wiring in the brain and the fluids that are also necessary to its operation. You know how irritable everyone becomes in an office if the air conditioning is not working on a hot summer's day. Everything else is O.K.—but that doesn't matter. If you're too hot, you can't work at top efficiency.

Then there are the people in the office. Each has a particular job necessary to the company's efficient operation. I have had a sketch of the brain drawn for you to look at as we develop our comparison of the brain to a business organization (Fig. 11). Miss Deep Brain will play our deep brain, Mr. Parietal our parietal lobe, Mr. Occipital the occipital lobe, Mr. Temporal, the temporal lobe and Mr. Frontal, the Chief Executive Officer or Big Boss, will play the frontal lobe, Mr. Legs and Miss Eyes are our legs and eyes.

As you enter the building, the first person you meet on the lower or first floor is Miss Deep Brain—the combination PBX operator and receptionist. She is possibly the lowest paid, yet in many ways the most important. If Miss Deep Brain doesn't do her job or if she's out sick one day, the whole company can be in an uproar. Phone messages may not be taken correctly or they may not be transmitted to the proper person. Since she also takes instructions from everyone else in the building (e.g. placing calls, seeing to it that one depart-

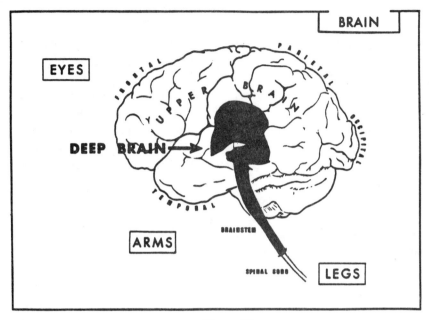

Figure 11.

ment's mail is relayed properly to another or directing a visitor to the right person), she must be able to take information and relay it properly.

On the other hand, if the wiring of her phone lines has been misconnected by the installation people, she can misdirect calls and not even realize what is wrong. Also, Miss Deep Brain can be the excitable sort of person who becomes confused with too much stress or work, and she just messes everything up despite her best intentions. So, incoming and outgoing visitors, phone calls and mail do not get handled properly in certain circumstances.

On the upper or second floor of this building besides Mr. Frontal, Big Boss, who has his office way up front, are the assistants who work for him, the Misters Parietal, Occipital and Temporal. Mr. Legs and Miss Eyes are workers in the field. Should Mr. Legs have an injury, he then must send a "pain" inquiry to Mr. Parietal asking if he is indeed hurting and where — thigh, knee, ankle — right or left? He must send this message through Miss Deep Brain who relays it to Mr. Parietal and sends his answer to Mr. Legs. "Yes, you have a pain in your right knee . . . you may now scream or cry!"

Should Miss Eyes see a tornado coming, she relays the sighting through Miss Deep Brain to Mr. Occipital for his analysis and interpretation. Mr. Frontal must weigh the information relayed to him for his judgment and make a decision about what to do. If Mr. Temporal who "polices" the building, in addition to other duties, is not feeling well, he might have Miss Eyes and Mr. Legs lose control, have a temper tantrum or even let all the other employees go berserk. However, if all employees are doing their job, the company responds to all information correctly and sends the message "take cover — tornado sighted."

Our brain must also be in "good" working order for life to go smoothly. If there are breakdowns in any part of it, problems surface. Jane, Ray, Marilyn, Sam, Jimmy, Butch, Carol and Steve all had problems with how their brain functioned — and all had problems coping with life.

We still don't know all we'd like to about the brain's functions. We know that the cortex is an operations center but is only part of the entire neurological system. The rest of the brain includes the nerve bundles or white matter that connect one part of the brain with another — back to front, side to side, up and down; the spinal cord and all the incoming and outgoing nerves that connect with the lower brain; and all the nerves that travel up and down the spinal cord with connections to every part of the body. It's quite a system! A malfunction anywhere can cause trouble.

For example, there may be a defective "wiring" connection between one specific part of the cortex and another specific part. The first part receives a message and can only process a part of it because that is its job and it doesn't "know" anymore. It must send the message on to the second part for further processing, but the connections to this area are down and not functioning. So the message is not processed further at this stage. This stage of the processing is bypassed. The final processing area gets an incomplete, even garbled, message and in essence says, "Hey, what's this stuff you're sending me? I can't handle it." Using visual associations as an example of a breakdown in brain processing, some children can easily recognize letters or words separately but not when embedded in a word or sentence. The processing network for this skill is not operating properly.

Though much more intricate, the electrical system of the brain is not totally unlike that which operates any appliance in your home. An electrician brings in a cable from the nearest power pole and service is available to you from your local power company. He then installs a circuit breaker box with all those confusing switches. After he has decided where all the sockets and switches should be, he pulls more wires from the box to the appropriate rooms and connects them where necessary.

It is not unusual, within your house, for a circuit to tie into several outlets or perhaps affect several rooms. So, if an extra appliance causes trouble, a whole area of the house may be without current until you disconnect that extra appliance that was the "straw that broke the camel's back." If overloading happens frequently, you can choose to have some rewiring done. To some degree, this is similar to what can happen in the brain.

A difference in your home's wiring and your brain's is that different parts of the brain's circuits mature at different times. A two-year-old cannot have the same degree of control over his balance or his behavior as a seven-year-old. It's not just a matter of size or physical maturation that makes it impossible for him to stand on one leg any length of time. He is neurologically unable to control his balance very long. Should the child, however, reach the age of seven and still not be able to stand on one leg, a delay or lag in maturation of the nervous system is usually given as the reason. Some investigators recently have questioned the concept of maturational lag. Rather, they consider these signs as defects in development. These defects remain but may be masked, overshadowed or compensated for by other new behaviors or skills which are made possible as the brain develops. The programmed development does go on leaving the defect behind!

Our brain is not fully developed at birth. We are not really all put together until final nerve connections are made in our twenties. If, in the meantime, there is some injury, some types of cells may repair themselves, but that is not always the case. Recovery may be in the form of another part of the brain taking over or substituting for the damaged portion. A person may again learn to speak in spite of a damaged speech center in the dominant, usually left, hemisphere of the brain. Nevertheless, "curative" measures may not be perfect. Another area may not make such a good substitute or damage may be only partially remedied. Inadequate repair may not be evident in persisting neurological signs but *only* in certain aspects of behavior or in certain circumstances. The number of "strategies" used to resolve problems may be reduced. In a classroom, a teacher gives a set of problems according to the grade level and expects the children to solve them. A child who has had a "repair job" may be unable to do so, and the frustration may result in a temper tantrum or behavior that the teacher perceives as unexpected or unexplainable — such as throwing a pencil across the room or a sudden burst of tears. These children may repeat the same error over and over, not understanding their mistake at the beginning. As they mature with uneven or incomplete development, some of their behavior may remain infantile or childish.

A good example of varying maturation rates in *parts* of the brain is obvious in teenagers. How often have you heard or said, "Johnny just doesn't have good sense!" The statement is not too far from wrong. The frontal lobe, which helps us consider the consequences of our actions, does not mature until the early twenties. Johnny is not likely to make the responsible decisions that would please his parents until that maturation takes place. It may be possible to help him arrive at a proper decision one time, but left to his own brain's devices, he may come up with a "spacey" response the very next time given the same problem. The result can be one speeding ticket after another, three "drunk" weekends or an allowance for a month spent in one day.

The glory of man is his ability to think. Temporary lapses in this ability are what people often mean when they say "use your head." In its role as organizer, director and final arbitrator of our responses, the frontal lobe is what makes this possible. It is somehow involved in all final decisions, right or wrong. It appears to supply our abstraction and synthesis abilities, our perception of relationships and differences, and the ability to deal with complex situations and to shift strategies. In short, it has the ability to plan or think out the next action. The entire frontal lobe has wide connections with all other lobes of the brain and the deep brain.

If, by chance, Johnny has "faulty wiring" between the frontal lobe and certain parts of the deep brain, he will be inflexible in his thought patterns. He will be almost incapable of switching from one kind of thought pattern to another. If he is asked to sort objects by shape, he can. But, if the next instruction is to sort them by color, he may be unable to do this. If two red shapes — a square and a circle — are placed together for him, he will place all other *square* pieces next to the red square or all *circles* beside the red circles. And, sorting by both color and shape is impossible. It is not his inability to form the original classification that is the problem: he cannot switch or let go of the first concept. He may think he has, but the results will show otherwise.

The frontal lobe system is not a single operation. Several parts of this lobe have a separate function and connect with other related areas of the brain. Injuries to a specific part of the frontal lobe may, as in Marilyn's case, relate to the inability to profit from information for any length of time. This appears to be due to distractibility, lack of attention to cues, or being "locked into" making the same error repeatedly.

Johnny may not be able to "chunk" or group-relate information. He cannot do problems requiring a series of steps and cannot analyze and synthesize patterns in complex pictures. Or, he cannot tell how many words are in a sentence or solve a word problem in arithmetic such as "how much is four plus four plus four?" He can be taught to chunk information by giving him longer spaces between words or phrases, color-coded words, written steps for solving arithmetic problems, etc. Sometimes, distractibility or restlessness is really the inability of Johnny's frontal lobe to carry out all the necessary actions for the successful completion of a plan or task. Johnny cannot sort out the successive steps to solve the problem.

In the normal brain, various strategies can be used at different times to meet specific circumstances; it is quite versatile due to the super-abundance of nerve connections or wiring. In the brain's attempt to meet all of life's challenges, it builds up a resource of options that work and eliminates the ones that don't. Ability and capacity continue to grow as the brain develops.

When the brain is damaged, some rewiring may occur. Various supporting elements or cells may transmit impulses around the "scar" site, but the dysfunctioned brain is still not well equipped. It can only use what is available.

Symptoms of brain dysfunction may not appear in a small child but only because he does not yet have the need for a particular brain circuit. This inadequacy may surface later as a learning or behavioral deficit when that particular part of the brain is needed. A child might indeed by an all "A or B" student in the first, second and third grade and may start making D's and F's when his brain is unable to handle the more complex problems of the fourth.

With all the interconnections between areas of the brain and the different rates of maturation, even a so-called *minor* dysfunction can compound the many difficult situations a child has to face. If dysfunction is present in the deep brain, it is somewhat like overloading our circuits. The deep brain makes it possible for the upper brain to organize our behavior in controlled and purposeful ways. It prepares or alerts the upper brain for action; it sifts through the many stimuli and selects those for processing. In fact, one part of the deep brain is called the reticular *activating* system. There might just be some truth to the saying: "I blew my top!"

In addition to the cortex of the brain and its system of connecting nerve bundles or "wiring" to its lobes and to the deep brain, it has yet another system: its brain chemistry. From just what has been uncovered recently, this system must be vast. We know something about a few of the enzymes and the neurotransmitters — produced by nerve tissue — and how they affect some aspects of behavior. One of the enzymes is monoamineoxidase. For easy reference, thank heaven, this has been shortened to "MAO." There appears to be an association between MAO and a variety of personality traits including gregariousness, high activity and a restless life-style. It has also been related to depression and inappropriate emotional reactions to circumstances.

MAO apparently influences behavior by breaking down the neurotransmitters that carry messages between nerve cells. By preventing a *buildup* of neurotransmitters, brain cells that probably would have been activated remain quiet. Lower MAO levels cause us to be very active and easily aroused. Some schizophrenics and depressives have low amounts of MAO in their brain chemistry. A study of newborns found that those with lower MAO levels were more excitable and crankier than others. It may be that MAO levels have a bearing on some types of behavior problems.

All the brain wiring and its enzymes and neurotransmitters make it possible for us to receive stimuli and give instructions to our body as to what to do. It is a very complicated, yet beautiful, communication system. It is in constant action—awake or asleep.

You can forget all the details about the brain, forget the business organization we compared it to, but do remember this: the brain must be in good working order or there will be trouble!

CHAPTER 7

FROM ONE EXTREME TO ANOTHER

ONE current belief about brain arousal proposes that the *hyperactive* child has abnormally low arousal — and the *hypoactive* child is really overaroused. While this appears to be backwards, let's take a look at the extremes in behavior.

One extreme example of an overaroused brain would be Kanner's syndrome. Most of you have heard of this by its popular name: autism. The foremost symptoms of this disorder are the inability to form social relationships and the obsession with keeping everything the same. If an autistic child is presented with something new (i.e. his routine is disrupted or changed), the reaction is catastrophic; he screams, thrashes, weeps. He may resort to self-damage, such as biting his own body.

It has been suggested that a chronically high and inflexible level of activity exists in the child's brain activating system. That is, there is always a high degree of arousal. To cope, the child will withdraw and exhibit other symptoms such as rocking, making faces, or exhibiting odd hand movements. As the situation becomes more stimulating, the movements become more profound. On the other hand, placed in a room by himself, the movements calm down.

This unusual behavior is apparently the child's way to prevent arousal levels from exceeding critical limits. He blocks further sensory input. For example, an autistic child is often suspected of being deaf but seldom tests out as having a hearing loss.

Another symptom found in the autistic child is an unusually high threshold for pain. This type of child appears not to feel stimuli pain-

58

ful to others and, consequently, will not react. It's possible that the extreme level of arousal blunts painful sensations.

Obviously, autism is an extreme in behavior types. But it's possible that the hypoactive child has a similar pattern. The seeming lethargy of the hypoactive child could be a means of reducing amounts of stimulation. This child may tire faster and be unable to work as long as the average student.

In their own particular ways, the hypoactive children are just as handicapped as hyperactive children. He or she is allowed to sit in class and waste away, deficient in academic and social skills. Because they are "such good children," they get litle attention. They usually have at least average intelligence, yet function below this level.

Another interesting observation in connection with the hypoactive child is that, even when excited or stimulated, the heart rate curve is essentially flat. Other children have a speeding up of heart rate, then the heart rate slows down. As with true hyperactives, the hypoactive child may show neurological signs of brain dysfunction as demonstrated on an EEG.

Our friend, Jane, shows most of the typical symptoms of hypoactivity. Her EEG did show abnormalities, and a blood test revealed a decrease in certain chemicals that should be in the brain fluids. Today, she is on medication which seems to be bringing some relief to chronic depression and an overreaction to her circumstances. She also continues therapy to learn new ways of behaving.

The hyperactive child's brain, according to the belief of this school of thought, is running around like crazy trying to find enough stimulation for himself. He is underaroused. He's the one who *should* study with the radio going. The additional stimulation actually helps him keep his mind on what he's doing. His erratic behavior, irritating as it is to those about him, is the result of his endless search for further stimulation.

A recent study in nerve physiology found that it is not only the brain cells that may be underaroused in hyperactive children. The nerve cells in the spinal cord responsible for movement were found to be *hypo*excitable or sluggish in response. The hyperactive child appears to have reduced ability to respond to rapidly delivered, repetitive stimuli and so he may need more of it to maintain adequate arousal.

Ray, obviously, typifies hyperactivity. Since he couldn't find enough legitimate activity on his own, he gradually became a serious problem and, eventually, became a legal problem for his parents and the community. With no help, it was an "anything goes" approach to create stimulation for himself. His EEG revealed a dysfunction, too.

If you go back through the cases I've described, you should be able to pick out the combination of signs in each that points to possible brain dysfunction. In these cases an EEG showed a pattern that verified an abnormality. There was a reason for each person to be as they were.

Since so much emphasis is put on hyperactivity, I thought I would discuss it in a little more detail. Actually, hyperactivity or the hyperactive syndrome, is now called attention deficit disorder with hyperactivity. This is because the inability to attend (that is, maintain vigilance and attention) is such a core feature of this disorder. The current view of hyperactivity plays down motor overactivity as defining symptoms in hyperactive children and stresses the greater importance of attentional deficits and impulsivity.

The American Psychiatric Association which has given us the term "attention deficit disorder" has a lengthy description of what goes into this diagnostic category in the latest edition of its *Diagnostic and Statistics Manual of Mental Disorders* (DSM-III). The list of symptoms under *Inattention* includes: fails to finish things he or she starts, often doesn't appear to listen, has difficulty concentrating on schoolwork or sticking to a play activity, etc.

Impulsivity is the inability to inhibit impulses (e.g. poor impulse control), which is translated by society into disobedience. Under *Impulsivity* are such descriptions as: often acts before thinking, shifts rapidly and excessively from one activity to another, has difficulty organizing work or awaiting turn in games or classroom, and frequently calls out in class.

Hyperactivity is the third group of symptoms listed under attention deficit disorder. It includes such descriptions as runs or climbs on things excessively, has difficulty sitting still or fidgets almost constantly, and is always "on the go" acting as if "driven by a motor." Other diagnostic points are that the onset of the disorder is before the age of seven and has been present at least six months.

There are less "official" lists of behaviors for the hyperactive or attention deficit disorder child. One list was made from the descriptions of parents and teachers. It has additional, and more specific, descriptions of behavior of the hyperactive in "down-to-earth" language. Some of these statements may fit your child: fiddles with things, talks incessantly, manipulates objects or body, interrupts, gets up and down during TV program or doing homework, requires adult supervision, has difficulty settling down for sleep, restless during travel, when taken shopping touches everything and restless during church, movies and while visiting relatives and friends.

Some investigators have cautioned us to understand that *increased* and *sustained* restlessness and motor activity is not "characteristic" of the majority of hyperactive children. Rather, it is the *eruption* of such activity (usually, in structured situations requiring impulse control) that typifies hyperactive children.

Recently, another important concept in our understanding of the hyperactive child has been published. It concerns a deficiency in *rule-governed behavior* or a child who lacks the ability to govern or rule himself. Parents and teachers see this as noncompliance. Rule-governed behavior refers to the control of behavior by words (verbal stimuli). Adults first provide these words externally in the form of commands and later they are "internalized" by the child. This is a kind of verbal regulation. However, the hyperactive child has difficulty internalizing or taking these words "onto his own." New studies, using neuropsychological test profiles, suggest that there may be functional abnormality of the left (verbal) brain in these children.

So, these are some of the things your attention deficit disorder child is made of: hyperactivity, noncompliance, poor self-control and poor at problem solving. If this describes your child or if you are a teacher and have such a child in your class, please get him help. Don't wait until he is fifteen and has "gone on" to "bigger and badder" behavior.

CHAPTER 8

BUT I AM TRYING!

HOW many times have parents and/or teachers said to a child: "You're not trying." The child responds: "But I am trying." The answer: "Try harder." Many of these children are telling the exact truth: they are trying but are unable to learn or to do what has been asked of them. They are damned if they do and damned if they don't — if they are learning disabled.

Don't get me wrong, there are some children who have problems at school and "learning difficulties" that are not related to brain dysfunction. A child's self-image, problems at home, disruptions in his life, such as death, divorce, or a move from familiar surroundings, can indeed lead to learning or behavioral problems at school or at home. These are not the children we want to identify.

Educators classify children as learning disabled if intelligence tests, or other measures of intellectual ability, result in scores that are at least in the average range but their performance is significantly below their ability in some or all subjects. Children with superior IQ's can still be learning disabled. A number of terms may apply to such contradictory information: brain-based learning disability and brain-related learning disability or the child may be referred to as a neurologically impaired learning disabled child.

The relationship between learning and behavior can show itself in several ways. There are children who like to learn and try but are often poor learners because of a short attention span. They can't keep their minds on the material long enough to learn it. Their brains cannot maintain or keep in operation the necessary learning circuits for the time needed to learn. They cannot attend to more than one thing at a time or shift their attention quickly from one thing to another.

For example, a child in the process of closing and putting away his book at the end of one lesson misses the instructions given during this process. At home, this child may well lose interest while you are reading him a story — you cannot keep his attention for any length of time. He does better on some days, worse on others. If tested, the child's EEG may show some type of abnormal activity such as epileptiform activity. These periodic disruptions in the electrical pattern interfere with adequate brain function. Or this child may have an immature EEG pattern, one that is expected in a much younger child.

Brain functions are not the same on both sides. The right brain takes care of our nonverbal or nonlanguage skills. It's the left brain that controls verbal and language abilities. Yet, for *many* nonverbal and verbal skills, the whole brain must be involved.

For example, if you see something standing upright, you only need the right brain. But, if the object is turned upside down, you need both sides to interpret what you see. There must be a consultation between the two sides to turn the object right-side up in the mind's eye in order to properly judge what you are seeing. The right brain can work out simple spatial tasks by itself; but add other abilities and the left brain must be called in for help. The more the verbal requirements, the more the left brain must participate.

It would seem that words, being verbal stimuli, would be totally managed by the left brain. But, when you realize that words are actually complex symbols, then you see that their processing must involve both sides.

Word recognition is a multi-stage process. The basic perceptual and spatial characteristics of the letters and words — the mechanics of reading and spelling — are handled by the right brain first. Then, the left brain supplies the meaning.

Students are often unable to give verbal reports of words they have visually matched. This indicates the different processes involved in matching and reporting. The whole cycle has not been completed. The current thinking, however, is that nonverbal skills aren't strictly a process of the right brain. They require both right and left brain. Verbal skills, however, appear to be much more the responsibility of the left brain.

In any brain rehabilitation unit you can see what brain dysfunction can do to skills. A sixty-year-old physician suffered a right brain stroke several months ago. He could not put together a simple seven-piece puzzle of a human hand — one of the easier items in a widely used intelligence test. He offered excuses and giggled, as many of us do when embarrassed, as he struggled to fit the third finger into the thumb position. He never could complete the puzzle correctly. He could formulate no organized plan as to how to go about it. He was in the position of an elementary school student who has right brain dysfunction. The child is expected to decode letters and work with puzzles and blocks and he simply cannot do this.

Studies have documented the advantage girls have over boys in the *early* mastery of abstract verbal reasoning and pattern matching skills. The boys, however, are superior on tests of spatial memory and motor skills. We know there is a difference in male and female brains. Since the methods for teaching reading and writing skills rely on verbal abilities, boys are in greater jeopardy than girls of developing learning disabilities because of their *normal* maturational skill deficiencies. Actually, in teaching such skills to boys, use should be made of their good spatial ability rather than relying solely on phonetics. Such sex differences are found to be more prevalent in kindergarten and less in second grade. Increasingly, requests are being made by parents for evaluation before entering their children in first grade. Some assessment at this time may provide information on which children might experience difficulty in the primary classes.

The school curriculum may create learning disabilities in children because of inherent developmental differences between boys and girls. But children who have a brain dysfunction will have problems with learning regardless of the curriculum. Hopefully, a preschool evaluation can tell which child has which problem.

As a child progresses in school, verbal skills become much more important. Learning disabilities may not become apparent until the middle primary school years. Nine- and ten-year-olds are sometimes found to have deficient comprehension and monitoring skills, both of which have a strong verbal base. Their difficulty does not appear to be simple inattention, impulsivity or memory limitations. These learning disabled children appear less able to process information they receive than normal children.

The ability to make accurate assessment of one's own level of comprehension is important in following instructions, listening to the teacher or following the presentation of the president of the company. If Johnny's comprehension and monitoring is adequate, he knows to question messages he doesn't understand. Billy, who cannot do this, is headed for great difficulty. We have methods now, and more are being developed, for training comprehension and monitoring skills. But we need to identify children who need this help.

A learning disabled child who is hyperactive or hypoactive is in even more trouble. It often takes them longer to process information. This may be part of the reason for their rapid loss of attention in the classroom. In turn, more errors are made. We have methods to help these children.

Studies of delinquent boys between the ages of fifteen and eighteen show that they had a verbal learning disability that followed them through school. While they performed on a par with other students insofar as motor abilities and simple skills were concerned, they showed severe impairment on highly verbal functions such as thinking and working through verbal concepts. They lacked a high level of perceptual organization, a level which requires much verbal input. These boys experienced consistent failure as a result of their deficits.

Follow-up studies of delinquent adolescents after five years found them still impulsive in a learning situation. They took less time to reflect over a solution to a problem when a number of alternatives were available. They were still weak in perceiving or understanding material independent of its context. These impulsive and hyperactive children were taught in the normal education programs without instructing them in the basics of successful problem solving. They had no help in learning impulse control or in learning to focus their attention.

The most common and perhaps the most disastrous specific learning disability for academic and occupational success is the inability to read well. Estimates range from 10 percent to 30 percent, depending on the classes sampled for the number of children who read significantly below their chronological and mental age. It is not unusual for these children to have difficulties in other areas. In both the global and more specific learning disabilities, the student may have low motivation for any learning experience. This can result from a number of failing experiences or from brain dysfunction.

There are almost as many theories about reading disabilities as there are reading disabled children. There is even a lack of agreement as to what terms to use. Some think that certain labels represent diagnosis by exclusion. Such a term, for example, is dyslexia. One gets the feeling that, all other causes of reading disability being eliminated, the unknown should be invoked: dyslexia. It is, unfortunately, an empty description and a disservice to the child. Despite the concerns of current investigators, dyslexia is a widely used term in referring to reading disabilities. It's difficult to tell, however, what is meant when it's applied to a given child.

It is believed that there are probably many forms of reading impairments. They may exist in varying degrees with other academic problems in math or spelling. They may coexist with a variety of other information-processing deficiencies in language and non-language areas. One does not cause the other, but the reading problem may be magnified by impaired processing skills in other areas.

Recent studies strongly suggest that learning disabled children are at much greater risk for conflict with society than normal children. In a two-year follow-up, it was found that boys with learning disabilities were three times as likely to be arrested for delinquent acts as other boys of the same age, social class and race. The largest increases in delinquency were among learning disabled boys whose parents had the highest levels of education and the most important occupations. It appears that the high expectations for success in such families made academic failure all the more crushing for these boys. They quickly followed the pressures from delinquent peers to escape and defy their families. Again, Ray is an excellent example of this behavior.

Professionals estimate that nine of every 100 boys in this country who have learning problems have been declared delinquent. Only four out of 100 boys in the population at large acquire this label. This does not take into account the unreported delinquent acts that have been "taken care of" and hushed up by family and friends. Findings like these seem to back up my belief that learning disabled children *must* be identified at an early age; otherwise, they may be heading for more problems than reading disabilities alone. There are personal and social consequences for the learning disabled other than delinquency. There are many unproductive or marginally productive lives that result from the inability to read, spell or write. These are the adults who have not had their chance to have a place in the sun.

For many teachers and parents, the term "dyslexia" means Johnny has average intelligence or better; he has had the opportunity to learn to read, but he still has difficulty. The academic use of the term, or diagnosis, is less general. It describes problems or "short suits" in language skills that make it difficult to read, write and spell. Common errors include reversals in letter writing: b for d, q for p, saw for was, quite for quiet, and many others. Sometimes there is an uncertainty as to right or left handedness, confusion about directions in space or time (that is, what is right and left, up and down, yesterday and tomorrow), along with arithmetic difficulties.

Desperate parents often hold the belief that their child cannot read well because he needs glasses. They hope that this will solve the problem. This idea has become so common that ophthalmologists have found it necessary to make a statement through their professional organizations. In it, they say that there is no peripheral eye defect that produces dyslexia and associated learning disabilities. They state that, with or without learning disabilities, the percentage of children with abnormal eyes is the same. Eye defects do not cause reversals in letters, words or numbers. The eyes are necessary for vision, *but the brain decodes or processes the information.* They point out that recent studies suggest dyslexia and associated learning disabilities may be related to genetic, biochemical and/or structural brain changes. Excluding correctable eye defects, glasses have no value in the treatment of dyslexia. In fact, unnecessarily prescribed glasses may delay needed treatment. They find no value in various eye exercises. Ophthalmologists urge early assessment and appropriate treatment of learning disabilities by educational and psychological specialists.

Many clinical psychologists and neuropsychologists believe that the source of reading and other learning disabilities is brain-related. For the present, little is known about how the brain accomplishes these feats, nor what has gone wrong in the brain that it cannot do these things. Most of us do not know how we learned to read. It just came naturally and rather early. So, it is difficult for us to understand why a child cannot read. Investigators speak of two broad forms of reading disability: a developmental or maturational reading disability, apparently due to slow or defective development of the brain, and an acquired reading disability not related to brain development.

Just as in motor impersistence, a three- or four-year-old is not expected to read like a seven- or eight-year-old. However, the older child should have some reading skills if his brain is developing normally. It is believed that developmental dyslexia accounts for only a small proportion of the total population of disabled readers.

Normally, the right-handed student has a larger visual region on the left side of the brain. Therefore, as we mature, the left hemisphere gradually assumes the reading and language functions. When there is a reversal of this situation, quite often the child is either a poor reader or cannot read at all. In one study, 40 percent of the reading disabled subjects showed this reversal. Some research proposes that such reversal results in language processing on a side of the brain that is not functionally suited to do this.

Researchers have stopped looking for just one cause of a reading disability. One child may have a visual-perceptual processing problem such as poor letter recognition, a right brain function; this is a visual-spatial dyslexia.

A reading disabled child may be found to have a verbal-linguistic problem. That is, his ability to process and organize words into meaningful thoughts, a left brain function, is impaired. Other recent work indicates that some reading problems may be due, to some degree, to poor communication between the right and left sides of the brain. Disabled readers may have difficulty moving the recognition of words to the language centers in the left brain — the area which categorizes and expresses what we experience. In these cases, the readers end up with misinformation or only a limited amount of the material actually read.

In the early grades the reading problem is more one of visual scanning and letter recognition. Reading disability surfaces in the later grades, mainly as a problem with comprehension. Some who have difficulty with word reproduction have intact recognition skills. They can detect their own or other's spelling errors despite their own poor visual imagery when attempting to reproduce a word.

Spelling disorders often accompany reading problems. However, they may be present on their own. As with reading disabilities, there are several types of spelling disorders; one has to do with difficulty in visual imagery. This is first visualizing a word, the hearing of the word, and finally pronouncing the word. There may be serial ordering and sequencing problems. This is the inability to reproduce letters and/or sounds in the correct order.

There is a rapidly developing area devoted to the study of how we think or what processes are used in thinking. This field of "cognitive psychology" speaks about two types of information processing: simultaneous and successive. In other words, we can think or process things simultaneously — in a grand sweep. Any part of the whole can be examined or extracted without going through the whole sequence or thought pattern in order. This is the basis, for example, of abstract thought as in formulating ideas or designs. The right brain is good at simultaneous processing.

The left brain contributes much to successive processing. There is a first step, second, third, etc. A simple example is bead-stringing from patterns or using the memory sequences of different-shaped beads. In fact, this is one of the tasks that has been used in tests of successive processing ability.

Children who show deficits in both abstract reasoning and sequencing memory (that is, a general language disability) read very poorly. Others may have good abstract reasoning yet be poor in verbal expression and memory. They are able to compensate for the deficits by using their good reasoning skills. Students with good sequencing-memory skills may develop a sight-word vocabulary, but their ability to comprehend an abstract meaning in what they read is impaired. They may retain isolated segments of information in short-term memory, but their inability to form concepts may limit long-term learning and retention. Naturally, those with the generalized deficit are the most difficult to remediate.

The ability to abstract — this is what real thinking is all about. It enables us to progress from the specific to the general and even soar beyond to produce new concepts. Abstraction involves the ability to plan. A high quality of thought requires mature functioning of the frontal lobes. Abstraction ability feeds on flexible thought patterns or the ability to switch lines of thinking and principles of action.

Four developmental stages specific to abstraction and frontal lobe function have been identified. In stage one the child merely describes activity in a disjointed fashion. Most normal children function at this stage at about two years of age.

In stage two there is still the inability to *switch* the principle of action. The child is actually neurologically incapable of switching or changing an action in progress, especially on verbal command. This is seen up to twenty-six months for simple tasks and for the first four years in tasks that involve more than one set of plans to be handled. A young child when intently engaged in a play pattern cannot switch to another activity because you have told him to do this.

In stage three, planning ability is seen. Finally, in stage four the beginnings of mature thought patterns emerge. Now the child can successfully switch the principle of an activity in progress. This happens by five years of age. Now your child has the ability to plan and to change plans if necessary.

Fascinating studies charting the development of abstraction ability and concept formation in young children have been reported. One group of studies used the narrative or story-telling technique in which children reconstructed stories told to them. By age five, less than 20 percent, were unable to show some ability to abstract material. Such findings are consistent with the known spurt in development of the various structures of the frontal lobe system taking place around the age of four.

The next spurt in frontal lobe function occurs during adolescence. Detailed investigations of juvenile delinquents using this narrative method turned up the finding that some of them do not have frontal lobe function sufficient enough for stage four, which is thought development. The ability to switch actions is not available to them. These delinquents may fall into criminal acts because of their inability to switch the principle or plan of an action in progress, to check for new solutions, and to compare these with the original intent. An innocent lark in a shopping mall may end up in shoplifting. A mere robbery might result in a killing when the owner of the house suddenly appears. This subgroup of juvenile delinquents may have other problems, but it is also their poor frontal lobe function which gets them into trouble.

An EEG study was done on a group of juvenile offenders. A significant number of them showed fontal lobe dysfunction in their EEGs (that is, the electrical pattern over the frontal lobes did not have the development expected for their age: it was immature).

The importance of recognizing the maturity level of thought and action patterns *should* be of first concern when dealing with certain delinquents and learning disabled school children. An eight-year-old child may do poorly in logical narration because he has the frontal lobe function of a four-year-old. There are practical rewards to society for helping the young student *to think*. Young persons whose frontal lobe system takes longer than two decades to develop show very high rates of arrest for serious crimes. These groups also have very high rates of fatal car accidents. The child who is unfortunate enough to have an unattended or unremediated deficit in abstraction ability is well represented in these groups.

Most parents have their own ideas about how their child is maturing—how he is learning and an overall "picture" of him. If these parents think that something is wrong and the problems appear to be similar to those of a child with a brain dysfunction, it is important to identify or rule out this possibility. Teachers and other professionals should also be concerned and at least discuss the subject with the parents.

CHAPTER 9

IT'S TIME FOR TESTING

So, the child needs, and is referred for, professional evaluation. What happens to him or her and to you? Well, many times there will be an EEG recommended or done. We've already discussed why this can be a very important part of the total testing procedure. Once in a while a CAT scan may be done. Then there is neurological testing for hard and soft signs, among other things.

Now comes the neuropsychological part. There are hundreds of psychological tests and many so-called "test batteries." Two neuropsychological batteries are the Halstead-Reitan and Luria-Nebraska. These are a collection of many different kinds of tests for memory, language, visual-perceptual ability, intellectual ability, etc. Emphasis is placed on the neurologic-type tests of nervous system functions — the motor abilities and visual, auditory, tactile and kinesthetic discrimination skills. One example of a kinesthetic test is to have the child close his eyes, then place the index finger over the middle finger. Kinesis skills are those which enable us to make simple and complex movements.

Examiners will vary in what tests and how many tests they use in their neuropsychological evauation. Perhaps a Bender Gestalt or other drawing test will be given. They may give tests or scales that you know as intelligence or IQ tests. The trick in this testing is not to focus on *a* score but to bring out or identify spared and impaired abilities. The best known of these types of tests are the Wechsler scales. There is the Wechsler Preschool and Primary Scale of Intelligence (WPPSI) for the four- to six-and-one-half-year old, and the

Wechsler Intelligence Scale for Children-Revised (WISC-R), which covers ages six through sixteen. The Wechsler Adult Intelligence Scale (WAIS) picks up from there. They give a verbal score derived from such subtests as Information, Vocabulary, and Similarities; and a nonverbal or performance score from Picture Completion, Block Design and Coding subtests. From these scores a Verbal IQ, Performance IQ, and Full Scale IQ is derived.

Another intelligence or cognitive ability test is the McCarthy Scales of Children's Abilities for age ranges two-and-one-half years to eight-and-one-half years. It gives a General Cognitive Index (GCI score) composed of scores for verbal ability, short-term memory, numerical ability, perceptual performance, and motor development. Items in the subtests include Counting and Sorting, Opposite Analogies, Tapping Sequence, Draw-A-Design, and Work Knowledge.

There is a new test just published which shows much promise. It is the Kaufman Assessment Battery for Children (K-ABC). This test is built around an actual concept of how the brain functions — the simultaneous and successive processing that we mentioned earlier. It can be used with children from two-and-one-half to twelve-and-one-half years.

In simultaneous processing there is an "all-together" or an "at-once" awareness — you look at the problem and immediately know the answer. Simultaneous processing tests are: Magic Window, Face Recognition, Matrix Analogies and Spatial Memory.

On the other hand, successive processing is dependent on serial order or succession. The material cannot be handled or solved at any one time. We put one bit of information after another in a certain order to get our answer, like a computer. Tests designed to measure successive processing include Photo Series, Hand Movements, Word Order and Number Recall. There is also an Achievement Scale which measures academic achievement — verbal fluency with Expressive Vocabulary and reading skills with Reading/Decoding and Reading/Comprehension. There are also Riddles, Arithmetic and Famous Faces and Places tests in the K-ABC.

The Kaufman tests may prove to be well suited for spotting spared and impaired abilities. An added plus is that remediation techniques based on this simultaneous-successive processing model are available. Once you have identified weakness in your child's learning abilities, you will be able to help your child at home.

Sometimes, in the neuropsychological assessment tests of reading ability may be recommended to find out specifics about a reading problem. There are tests, such as Illinois Test of Psycholinguistic Abilities (ITPA), which give information on several aspects of reading and language skills such as auditory closure, sound blending, visual sequential memory, etc. Another test is the Boder Test of Reading-Spelling Patterns which is a diagnostic screening test for subtypes of reading disability.

The testing is now behind you and your child. What now? The neuropsychologist has had an opportunity to see the child in action and the test results and may even have done part of the testing. He or she has asked critical questions of the parents who brought the child (e.g. have other members of the family had reading problems, were they hyperactive, etc.?). Ideally, the professional who is in charge of the assessment can also interpret the EEGs. That way, what is found in the EEG as it rolls off the machine can be related to the neuropsychological findings on the spot. The EEG can be shown to the parents, who then are better able to understand the connection between Johnny's brain wave pattern and his learning or behavior problems. The results of the other tests are also reviewed with the parents. The implications of the findings are discussed and ways of dealing with the situation are suggested and planned. This type of session, really a combination assessment and counseling session, is helpful and reassuring.

No parent need be frightened of this kind of testing. It is not painful and can be fun for a child. You can be reassured that there is no "pass-fail," only information you need to know about your child.

CHAPTER 10

THE SOONER THE BETTER

IT is never too soon to look carefully at your child and to make an honest evalation. Try to remember what this child was like in the crib (restless and agitated, nothing pleased him) or was he or she quite unresponsive (not really caring if you were there or not, not smiling or cooing when you approached).

Mothers of hyperactive children often notice that there is something unusual about their child early in infancy. In one investigation, half of the mothers of hyperactive children remember feeling that their children were different before their first birthday. These mothers commonly reported that their hyperactive children were very active in the crib, climbed out of playpens early, and have been running ever since they could walk. These children also have had feeding, sleeping and general health problems more often than normal children.

Another study on infant temperament and development found that boys with severe learning problems as infants were lower in activity level, more irregular in habits, and less approaching and negative in mood than normal boys. This is the boy seen later in school as the hypoactive slow learning child. They are the infants who even in their cribs were characteristically slow to respond. They had a low activity level, did not smile or cuddle very easily, had low approach, were irritable, low in mood and inconsistent or unpredictable in their habits.

These characteristics are also likely to have an impact on a parent. These infants could have a dampening effect on maternal behavior. The mother's involvement with the infant may diminish as she is not *rewarded* by the child with a smile as she cuddles and talks to the infant. At the other extreme of behavior, hyperactive children also may have an effect on the parents because of their less intense personal or social bonds. They are usually less person-oriented than the average children. They appear not to need people contact and even in the crib seem not to care if anyone approaches or not.

Much study has gone into the effects of the parents on the child but little on the effects of the child on the parent. The child who is not very verbal, or appears disinterested, is reacted to differently, often negatively, by the mother or father who happens to be very verbal and outgoing. The linguistic level of the child controls the adult verbal responses to the child and even spreads to the nonverbal responses, such as hugs and kisses.

This reciprocal impact of parents and infants is a topic that is in the early phases of study. We need a better understanding of infant-parent impact and what happens in the early childhood years to increase the risk of such a child developing a learning disability or a conduct problem. It is also important to the well-being of the parent. Many a family has been broken up, or their lives and behavior changed, by a child who is hyperactive, unpredictable, low in people interest, irritable, not communicative, lethargic, or an early conduct problem among family and friends. Sadly, parents often berate themselves or feel guilty over their feelings or how they react to their child, when in fact they were responding to the abnormal behavior of their child. It takes courage to ask, "What is the kid doing to us?"

It is known that more abused children are hyperactive, or have other behavioral problems, than the nonabused. But on the other side of the coin are the parents who have been abused and/or physically attacked by their offspring. Such early childhood histories can be very helpful to the preschool teacher by alerting her to watch certain children for signs of developing behavior and learning problems. Yet, many parents are too embarrassed to share this information with teachers or even the child's doctor.

The importance of early histories is highlighted in a study of children with a history of accidental poisoning (particularly the repeaters) and hyperactivity. In a first grade group of children, over 20 percent of the hyperactive boys had been accidentally poisoned, but only 6 percent of the boys who were not hyperactive. The poisonings occurred between ages one and six years. One-half of the repeaters had one or more siblings who had also been accidentally poisoned, and over one-half of the families with repeaters had other children with major behavior problems.

The descriptions of the children hospitalized for accidental poisoning are most revealing. They were described as daredevils, overactive, impulsive, being into things all the time, and an overall behavior problem. Other descriptions included hyperactivity, distractibility, temper tantrums, and disobedience.

Now, look at how your child is doing in nursery and preschool. How does the child mingle socially? Children with low social competence are the children who keep to themselves, 'fail to play with other children, do not take part in activities unless urged, have a downcast expression, seldom smile, and appear to stare blankly into space. Also at risk for problems later is a child who does not conform to the standards of society. He or she gets angry when an adult interrupts his play even though this is a normal routine, such as suppertime or bedtime. He or she dislikes other children and shows deliberate cruelty to them (e.g. bullies, hits and picks on them). This child screams and bangs objects when angry, is easily irritated or frustrated, fails to obey or follow instructions or directions of an adult, or "talks back." The child gets angry or annoyed when talked to by an adult, even when this is in a friendly manner and not a reprimand. It is important to the child that you observe and *note* these behaviors. However, not all of these children will be brain dysfunctioned, but some will be.

It is important that children at risk for behavior and learning problems be identified as soon as possible. And we always can use more information. It is not unusual now to see research papers on the *early* identification of behavior problems and learning disabilities and detection of brain dysfunction. These studies were done on preschool children and younger. Before this concentrated research effort was made, almost all children with these problems were usually called "socially immature," when, in reality, some of them were laboring under the whims and dictates of a brain not functioning normally. It's a tough situation for such a child to meet alone when no one recognizes that he cannot control his behavior.

Some of the preschool investigations have become very sophisticated. "Conceptual tempo" refers to the ability of children to regulate their thinking to meet changing situations; that is, changing levels of complexity in a task or changing sets of instructions.

Children who have difficulty changing pace or "conceptual tempo" appear to be at high risk for learning disability. An example would be that they are less able to alter tempo or course when going from simple to complex situations such as when told to work fast or to work slow. They cannot "change gears" when asked to walk fast, then walk slow. The child's inability to change with the situation can further be demonstrated with a simple drawing task. Children are asked to draw a straight line down the middle of a one-inch wide pathway drawn vertically on a long piece of paper. When asked to draw in the pathway "as fast as you can" and then told to "take as much time as you need," these high-risk children had difficulty in changing speed or "tempo."

Of course, formal psychological tests can be given the preschool youngster. For example, preschool children who do well on the drawings of the Bender Gestalt have been found to have better achievement scores after a year of primary school than the children who do poorly on this test. But one can also gain some information about academic ability and readiness from the simple circle, square, etc. drawings already shown in Figure 9.

Recognizing potential language problems can be noted by simply listening to your child. Many teachers of preschool children do just that: note the child's language.

Children who follow a normal course of development tend to use two-word sentences by two years of age. Children with developmental language problems, on the average, are three-and-one-half before they use two-word sentences. When once speaking in sentences, these language-delayed children use many of the same grammatical structures as do normal children, but they produce sentences with parts omitted. These are frequently the smaller words such as prepositions and conjunctions resulting in a language that is *telegraphic*. Verbs are particularly difficult for the language-disordered child, especially the verb forms *is* and *are*, *was* and *were*. Comparing normally speaking three-year-olds with language-disordered six-year-olds, few differences were found between the two groups. This suggests that after the language-disordered child reaches a certain stage of linguistic development, the language skills become fixated at this level. Unless the child receives help, his progress is very slow.

When preschool children who are acquiring language in a normal manner and rate are asked to desribe a common object, they not only give its name but also information about the object, its characteristics, and how you use it. Children of the same age with a language problem may also give the object's name. However, they are unable to elaborate and give additional information.

Children who are language impaired are likely to have problems with symbols or words which represent a concept or idea. They also have difficulty altering word forms or in using the tenses — past, present and future. An example would be a child who says "yesterday I walk" but omits the past tense of the verb walk. When a four- to six-year-old talks this way consistently ("baby talk"), he may have a language disability.

So we have many things we can look for in young and preschool children: their behavior, how they act in groups, how they perform in school, how they do on little tests, and how their speech is developing. If you spot trouble signs, you might consider a professional evaluation before your child enters first grade. You can make certain he is "ready" to enter school. Many schools have evaluations, but unfortunately, a child usually has to "fail" first.

CHAPTER 11

HELP! HELP! WHO OR WHAT CAN HELP?

NOTE that the chapter heading says help, not cure. Now, (and it is about time) professionals are talking about doing what they can to improve the child's impaired skills, but the emphasis is on beefing up the skills which are not defective rather than spending precious time trying to bring the impaired skills up to academic standards. There is now acceptance on the part of many educators that some child may have permanent limitations in some academic skills. Some Johnny may never be made into a good reader regardless of "remedial reading," but he could be developed into a darn good listener.

Professionals working with hyperactive children write books for other professionals such as Dr. Russell Barkley's *Coping with Hyperactive Children and Adolescents*. Throughout the book, he stresses that hyperactivity cannot be cured and that the rule in the treatment of hyperactive children is periodic "interventions" designed to *improve* the disorder. The restless, impatient and easily angered child becomes the restless, impatient and easily angered adult. But, as children, they may be given coping skills — that is, taught how to meet and handle themselves in certain situations.

Now that we have made that clear, there are various things that can be done. One of the first stops for many children with a behavior problem is your physician. He may use the EEG test to determine what, if any, medication may be best for your hyperactive child. Studies have shown that some hyperactive children have an epileptiform pattern in their EEG. Some have an immature EEG, rhythms

80

or patterns too slow for age, and characteristic of a younger child. The stimulant medications can be particularly effective in hyperactive children with such an EEG pattern. For some reason, this type of medication increases the frequency of the basic brain rhythm to nearer age level, and with this change, comes an improvement in hyperactivity and aggression.

The EEG can be used not only to record but to improve brain function. It is a physiological method which has received some attention and refinement in the last few years. In some cases EEG biofeedback, as it is called, can "train" the brain to produce certain rhythms. It may make the brain produce more and better alpha rhythm, which is the basic frequency of the normal brain. It has been reported that some learning disabled school children with this type of training have been able to do better in some subjects, such as arithmetic.

Another form of brain wave training is SMR biofeedback. SMR stands for sensorimotor rhythm. It is a rhythm of a certain frequency (14 cycles per second) picked up in certain locations on the scalp which can suppress some types of abnormal electrical activity; no one knows why. The brain is trained to increase its output of SMR in certain situations. Some successes have been reported in reducing the activity level and increasing the attention span in hyperactivity. It may be used at first in combination with medication and the medication tapered off as the training continues.

The educators have been busy devising instructional aids for the learning disabled child; some of these you are familiar with. Before helping Johnny to read, it is well to try to find out "why Johnny can't read." Is it one of the visual-spatial deficits such as an "embedding" or reversal problem or an auditory-verbal comprehension difficulty?

There are many ways to aid your learning impaired child. Here are a few examples.

For young children who are developing language and reading skills, help is given by the good old methods familiar to the parent. The child is drilled to make associations between visual material, such as pictures and designs, and the letters or words to be learned — the alphabet cards with pictures and picture-word matching which help the child build a reading vocabulary. There are also color-coded reading aids which focus the child's attention on specific words, word forms and phrases. Reading-impaired children with difficulties in both auditory (hearing) and visual (sight) processing might benefit from reading through writing methods — a child reads and writes at the same time. This type of exercise reinforces the visual-auditory associations by the muscle feedback associated with the act of writing.

The children who reverse letters can be given a set of letters to work with which cannot be reversed. The child whose only problem is producing mirror images can be given a felt board to work on. If he attempts to flip the letters over, he will be putting them on the board with the felt side up and they will fall off. The child should be shown why they fall off. In most cases, the child will also write letters upside down. This requires work with a special board, one on which the letters can be attached to the board only on one side and in only one place. A board with metal strips for lines and a small magnet at the top back of each letter does well. Rotating or flipping letters will make the letters fall off the board.

Before these procedures are started, see if the child can be taught to write script rather than printing. Script letters, because of their shapes and the flow of their beginning and end strokes, are much less ambiguous than printed letters. Many of the milder reversal problems are noted to disappear around the time that the writing of script letters is introduced. In fact, some school systems as in Ireland start the child writing with script letters and do not go through the printed letter phase. Teachers in these schools report much fewer reversal problems when writing is taught this way.

Some children with right brain dysfunction can identify letters or words when they are by themselves but cannot deal with these same letters or words when they are part of a sentence. These children cannot handle *embedded* material which is one of the skills needed in reading. There are drills which can be used for practice on *extracting* words from sentences and specific shapes such as circle, triangle, etc. from a design.

Many of these remediation aids can be purchased from one of the teacher supply houses. Ask your child's teacher about this. You can work with your child alone or with other parents who are in the same boat.

With spelling problems, the usual approach is merely to correct the wrong spelling. There are better ways to help a child with spelling. These methods use *error awareness*, making use of, or developing, the child's recognition skills. Also, this method helps the attention problems which many of these children have. Seeing a demonstration of the incorrect spelling of a word and then the correct way, the child focuses on the differences between the wrong spelling and the correct one. There are many variations and extensions of this technique.

Your child, even with intensive help, may never have good non-verbal skills. Often, these children have good left brain function. They are very verbal and language-sensitive. In the early grades, emphasis is placed on the nonverbal or nonlanguage skills. For these learning disabled children, you might help them develop their language skills early. This child may remain reading impaired because of chronic perceptual deficits, but this poor reader can compensate or cope by being made into a good listener. Teachers and parents can develop the child's skills by having him listen to taped stories, directions and explanations. Parents can prepare their own tapes on any and all subjects and there are also packaged programs which can be purchased, even for the first grade. When test time comes around, the child should be given the opportunity to take some tests orally.

There are children who have learned to decode letters and words, but they lack a comprehension or understanding of what these words and phrases mean in a sentence, a left brain task. Children with left brain dysfunction may have problems with verbal material for other reasons. They just do not learn well by listening to someone. They have difficulty visualizing and understanding material which is presented verbally. They stumble around looking for the right words to express what they are thinking. Often they do well, even superior work, at the nonlanguage level. If remediation is unsuccessful, these children should be made to feel comfortable with their deficit. It is alright to demonstrate, illustrate and draw their way through life. And now in this age, we have many visual aids such as video tapes and computer programs, and there are jobs that do not require a person to write or talk well.

There is a rapid developing area of remediation for learning impaired children who do not know how to think. They have poorly organized thinking strategies; they cannot solve problems. This area of instruction is called cognitive education.

One of the techniques used in cognitive remediation is focused or preorganized instruction. The focusing technique is a simple one, reading stories to the child. Good narrative stories and folk tales, such as those from Hans Christian Andersen, are read individually to a child. The child is asked to give what he or she remembers about the story. It is best to tape the responses. Here is where the focusing comes in. Before the story is read, the child is instructed to watch for certain things in the story and to focus on three things: the problem, how it was solved and the lesson to be learned from the story. The actual reading of the story is broken into three parts corresponding to the focused points. Each part is introduced by the comment, "Now, in this part watch for. . . ." Talk to the child about his version of the story. See if he understands what the story is all about. Ask if there is a moral to the story, such as honesty is the best policy or what the child learns from the story. Discuss other possible endings. You are helping your child learn to think. Even for normal children, educators now suggest that school should teach children *how to think* rather than having them learn just "facts and figures" that often become outdated.

Now, we come to how the psychologist and his work might help a child with a behavior problem. We are always being reminded that there are no problem children but only children with a problem.

You were told that two of the components of hyperactivity or attention deficit disorder are: impulsivity (lack of normal controls) and the inability to internalize rules and commands. A very simple principle can be used with these children. Have the child instruct himself—self-instruction! How does one do this?

One simple self-instruction technique uses a children's pencil maze. One is illustrated in Figure 12. This method incorporates the THINK ALOUD principle. It is a "talking through" method, first aloud, then whispering, and finally "talking to oneself" internally. The child tries to complete the maze without his pencil crossing or bumping into the lines of the pathways. The child is encouraged to talk out loud and to tell himself what to do, such as: "not too fast now—go slow here—be careful at this curve. Look, I'm finished. I did it with only one mistake!" A child who can eventually master the ability to talk to himself can police his own actions—can tell himself what to do. A variety of these mazes can be purchased at teacher supply houses.

Many classrooms in the lower grades have self-instruction or self-command cards and posters, for example: STOP in big letters or

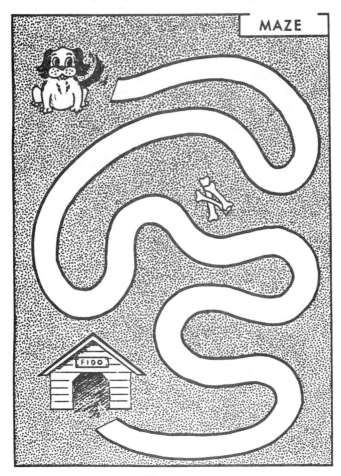

Figure 12.

SLOW-LOOK and phrases such as THINK BEFORE I ANSWER. The cards can be held up or laid on the table and pointed to when needed. Spoken words can be substituted in some cases (e.g. "Michael think") said at the proper time. Simple hand signals, such as the hand signal indicating stop, are also used. These cues, the spoken "Michael think" and the visual hand signal, can be used in combination by the teacher when Michael is seen leaving his seat, talking without permission or being rowdy and disruptive. STOP, LISTEN, LOOK and THINK posters are now a common sight in classrooms. These can be used at home.

Training in self-instruction or self-directed verbal commands can be used with preschool children who may need such a program before they enter the first grade. This training could be expanded by the first grade teacher. For example, the child tells himself: Go directly to the pencil sharpener in the front of the room and back again without stopping to talk, tease, or touch other children along the way.

There are yet other versions of this basic self-instruction method. The self-control principle is used with aggressive and hyperactive children in one of the THINK ALOUD programs. This program starts with exaggerated modeling or copycatting techniques. Then the child is encouraged to verbalize, or say out loud, the way he would solve a problem. He finally learns to do this without having to talk out loud—he listens to his inner voice. It has been successful with some children in improving their social behavior and school work. If you are interested, ask someone who is familiar with this program.

Still other variations of self-instruction are found in self-management training. Children are taught to correct their own work. They are taught how to use an answer guide to check their completed work such as their math problems and to give themselves one point for each correct answer. Eventually, the children check their own math work in their *own* classrooms. They total the number they got right, correct wrong answers and add up the points they earned or their score. Their math often improves and so may their work in other areas such as reading. They are learning to pay closer attention to what they are reading and will correct their own mistakes.

In addition to improving schoolwork, training in self-instruction and self-correction may improve the child's social behavior. This filters down as an increased responsibility for one's own failure. Control over his *own* outcome is in his own hands—whether doing schoolwork or getting along with other children or just learning how "not to get in trouble."

I have given you a few examples of remediation methods and training techniques—things to do that can help a child learn or help a child *learn* to behave. Many are easily used at home and are inexpensive, such as the self-instruction cards. Some offices and businesses are even using these to remind their employees TO THINK, PLAN AHEAD, or even TURN OFF THE LIGHT. These can be a fun way to teach at home.

CHAPTER 12

WHERE DO WE GO FROM HERE?

L EARNING is basic to the good life. True, learning impairment is not life-threatening, but it is a handicap which can result in a serious loss of human potential. A learning or behavior problem can spread to so many other areas of a person's life. This is especially significant in our society, which is so dominated by technological advances, that the ability to learn is more important than ever.

More and more educators are doubting the notion that children's learning problems will self-remediate. They are coming right out and saying that they no longer believe that "if we'd just be patient and give these kids enough time they can outgrow anything!" They see children who have problems in kindergarten, and these children have the same problems five years later. They are now asking if a child's learning problems appear to be chronic. Will it remain the same no matter how much remediation is given in the lower grades? This is a legitimate question. There are learning deficits that we just do not know how to improve yet. It may then be a matter of accepting the deficit — or problem. Then we will be free *early* to work with the child's strong skills and develop these.

The long-term studies on children with behavior problems are now coming in. These children were followed from infancy through adolescence, and even into early adulthood. Many of them either retain their initial problems or develop modified or new ones. Irritable, hyperactive, and difficult-to-manage toddlers are the same children with behavior problems in elementary grades. The solution is to teach these children coping skills.

Let me tell you about a study on an unusual group of air force cadets. These sixteen young men were referred to a psychiatrist because they had difficulty performing the basic tasks of military training. They found it difficult to learn how to march properly and how to fold and arrange various clothing items and equipment — something you must do in the service. In general, their ability to learn new motor type tasks, such as formation drills and judo techniques, were inferior to those of the other members of their squad. Besides these problems, these students showed marked irritability and anxiety. Some complained that they had great difficulty concentrating. Even so, some of them were highly motivated and wished to continue with their air force careers.

It was found that many of these cadets had always been considered "sloppy" by their families. In childhood they had difficulty in making their beds, folding their clothes neatly, keeping their toys arranged. Usually a member of the family would help them with their chores. It was found that fourteen of them had a history of temper tantrums as a child and were described by their mothers as being easily frustrated. Twelve had a history of hyperactivity which tended to disappear at adolescence. Ten of the students had speech problems which disappeared with age.

In secondary school these individuals did seem to get along with their peers. However, their histories clearly show that these students had avoided areas where a high degree of perceptual-motor skill was needed; they compensated by developing devious personality traits such as a "talent" for getting other people to handle jobs that they could not do. As they grew up, their difficulty seemed to "disappear" until they were thrust into a situation (air force) which demanded a high level of visual-motor ability and their problems reappeared. It was at this time that they developed symptoms which resulted in a referral to a psychiatrist.

The investigators who wrote the report cautioned that not all deficits associated with brain dysfunction have a spontaneous remission as had been generally believed in the past. The retained deficits surface when optimal performance is required or when more is asked of the person. The authors of this report said that a diagnosis or a precise label is less important than to understand the spared and impaired skills of the student and the way in which he or she learns and functions. By knowing his own abilities, a student is able to make realistic plans for his career or job. Don't be a mechanic if you can't handle tools. Don't be an accountant if you cannot do math (but maybe *you* can be a mechanic).

I don't like to use the words brain dysfunction any more than you do, but it is a very real fact of life for some children. The name of the game is identify and understand. Recall what happened in my cases that I told you about. Sure, some people manage to cope or compensate successfully, *on their own*, with a brain dysfunction that they are not even aware they have.

People may have brain dysfunction and never have to seek professional help because, in their case, the particular brain circuits involved are not critical to the skills they use to make a living or to get along in society. In reality, no handicap exists for them. Others cannot do this — not without help.

Now for a story with a good ending. I happened to be listening to CBS News on August 24, 1982. You might recall that after the fall of Saigon, a planeload of Vietnam orphans were being flown to parents here who had adopted them. The door of the plane blew out at a very high altitude, rapidly depressurizing the cabin and exposing these children to low oxygen levels. They were the victims of anoxia. One of the fathers appeared on the program and told about his son's learning difficulties and behavior problems. He said that many of the children on that plane had the same problems. They were getting help though — in their cases through our government. In fact, these children and their parents have gatherings every year in Washington to see how they are all doing and to compare notes. Many of them are better. The key is early detection (easy in this situation) and early help.

So, all is not gloom and doom. A new day is coming. New methods for helping children are coming from current psychological and educational research. And, even better detection techniques are likely in the near future. There is the rapidly growing, almost unbelievable, research into the chemistry of the brain, such as the neurotransmitters and enzymes. Help may come from this area at any time. But let us use *now* what we know about detecting learning and behavior disabilities and brain dysfunction; let us teach the coping skills or use other methods of teaching. Help these children now, don't wait.

BIBLIOGRAPHY

Barkley, Russell A. *Coping with Hyperactive Children and·Adolescents: A Handbook for Diagnosis and Treatment*. New York, The Guilford Press, 1981.

Campbell, Susan B., Endman, Maxine W., and Bernfield, Gary. A three-year follow-up of hyperactive preschoolers into elementary school. *Journal Child Psychology Psychiatry, 18*:239-249, 1977.

Camp, Bonnie W., Bloom, Gaston E., Herbert, Frederick, and van Doorninck, William J. "Think aloud": A program for developing self-control in young aggressive boys. *Journal of Abnormal Child Psychology, 5*:157-169, 1977.

Corkin, Suzanne. Serial-ordering deficits in inferior readers. *Neuropsychologia, 12*:347-354, 1974.

Cunningham, Mark D., and Murphy, Philip J. The effects of bilateral EEG biofeedback on verbal, visual-spatial and creative skills in learning disabled male adolescents. *Journal of Learning Disabilities, 14*:204-208, 1981.

DeFries, J.C., Singer, S.M., Foch, T.T., and Lewitter, F.I. Familial nature of reading disability. *British Journal of Psychiatry, 132*:361-367, 1978.

Dunleavy, Raymond A., and Baade, Lyle E. Neuropsychological correlates of severe asthma in children 9-14 years old. *Journal of Consulting and Clinical Psychology, 48*:214-219, 1980.

Durfee, Kent E. Crooked ears and the bad boy syndrome: Asymmetry as an indicator of minimal brain dysfunction. *Bulletin of the Menninger Clinic, 38*:305-316, 1974.

Jurko, M.F., and Andy, O.J. Post-lesion yawning and thalamotomy site. *Applied Neurophysiology, 38*:73-79, 1975.

Kinsbourne, M., and Warrington, Elizabeth K. The development of finger differentiation. *Quarterly Journal of Experimentl Psychology, 15*:132-137, 1963.

Krynicki, Victor E. Cerebral dysfunction in repetitively assaultive adolescents. *The Journal of Nervous and Mental Disease, 166*:59-67, 1978.

Lambert, Nadine M., and Sandoval, Jonathan. The prevalence of learning disabilities in a sample of children considered hyperactive. *Journal of Abnormal Child Psychology, 8*:33-50, 1980.

Lubar, Joel F., and Shouse, Margaret N. EEG and behavioral changes in a hyperkinetic child concurrent with training of the sensorimotor rhythm

(SMR). *Biofeedback and Self-Regulation, 1*:293-306, 1976.

Maier, Arlee S. The effect of focusing on the cognitive processes of learning disabled children. *Journal of Learning Disabilities, 13*:34-38, 1980.

Masterson, James F. The symptomatic adolescent five years later: He didn't grow out of it. *American Journal of Psychiatry, 123*:1338-1345, 1967.

McLeod, John, and Greenough, Pauline. The importance of sequencing as an aspect of short-term memory in good and poor spellers. *Journal of Learning Disabilities, 13*:255-261, 1980.

Meichenbaum, D.H., and Goodman, J. Training impulsive children to talk to themselves: A means of developing self-control. *Journal of Abnormal Psychology, 77*:115-126, 1971.

Miccinati, Jeannette. Teach reading disabled students to perceive distinctive features in words. *Journal of Learning Disabilities, 14*:140-142, 1981.

Miller, John W., and McKenna, Michael. Disabled readers: Their intellectual and perceptual capacities at differing ages. *Perceptual and Motor Skills, 52*:467-472, 1981.

Milman, Dorris H. Minimal brain dysfunction in childhood. Outcome in late adolescence and early adult years. *Journal of Clinical Psychiatry, 24*:371-380, 1979.

Morrison, James B., and Minkoff, Kenneth. Explosive personality as a sequel to the hyperactive-child syndrome. *Comprehensive Psychiatry, 16*:344-347, 1975.

Offord, D.R., Sullivan, K., Allen, N., and Abrams, N. Delinquency and hyperactivity. *The Journal of Nervous and Mental Disease, 167*:734-741, 1979.

Paulsen, Karen A., and O'Donnell, James P. Relationship between minor physical anomalies and "soft signs" of brain damage. *Perceptual and Motor Skills, 51*:402, 1980.

Ponitus, Anneliese A., and Ruttinger, Katherine. Frontal lobe system maturational lag in juvenile delinquents shown in narrative test. *Adolescence, 11*:509-518, 1976.

Richman, Lynn C., and Lindgren, Scott D. Patterns of intellectual ability in children with verbal deficits. *Journal of Abnormal Child Psychology, 8*:65-81, 1980.

Riddle, K. Duane, and Rapoport, Judith L. A 2-year follow-up of 72 hyperactive boys. Classroom behavior and peer acceptance. *Journal of Nervous and Mental Disease, 162*:126-134, 1976.

Rosenberg, John B., and Weller, George M. Minor physical anomalies and academic performance in young school children. *Developmental Medicine and Child Neurology, 15*:131-135, 1973.

Rubin, Rosalyn, and Balow, Bruce. Infant neurological abnormalities as indicators of cognitive impairment. *Developmental Medicine and Child Neurology, 22*:336-343, 1980.

Shelley, Edward M., and Riester, Albert. Syndrome of minimal brain damage in young adults. *Diseases of the Nervous System, 33*:335-338, 1972.

Surwillo, Walter W. Changes in the electroencephalogram accompanying the use of stimulant drugs (Methylphenidate and Dextroamphetamine) in hyperactive children. *Biological Psychiatry, 12*:787-797, 1977.

Von Hilsheimer, George, and Kurko, Virginia. Minor physical anomalies in exceptional children. *Journal of Learning Disabilities, 12*:462-469, 1979.

Waldrop, Mary Ford, and Halverson, Charles F., Jr. Minor physical anomalies and hyperactive behavior in young children, 343-380. In J. Hellmuth (Ed.): *Exceptional infant: studies in abnormalities*, Vol. 2. New York: Brunner/Mazel, 1971.

Waldrop, Mary F., Bell, Richard Q., and Halverson, Charles F., Jr. Newborn minor physical anomalies predict short attention span, peer aggression and impulsivity at age 3. *Science, 199*:563-564, 1978.

Weiss, Gabrielle; Minde, Klaus; Werry, John S.; Douglas, Virginia; and Nemeth, Elizabeth. Studies on the hyperactive child. VIII. Five-year follow-up. *Archives General Psychiatry, 24*:409-413, 1971.